A Year
on Planet
Alzheimer

and a little longer in Canada

By

Carolyn Steele

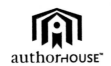

authorHOUSE™

1663 LIBERTY DRIVE, SUITE 200
BLOOMINGTON, INDIANA 47403
(800) 839-8640
WWW.AUTHORHOUSE.COM

First published by AuthorHouse 10/07/04

ISBN: 1-4184-9838-6 (sc)

Printed in the United States of America
Bloomington, Indiana

This book is printed on acid-free paper.

Artwork for cover by Reagan Thorne

To Zuscha,

who could teach us all a thing or two.

Acknowledgement

Everybody deserves a thank-you, each and every individual in the following pages without whom there would never have been an escapade. I'd like to add a few people whose names don't appear anywhere else though, for without their kind encouragement there would never have been a book:

Anna who first published my 'Letters from Canada' in London Mensa News and kept asking for more.

Miranda and Emma and the rest of the Rough Guides team, who were kind enough to accept snippets for 'proper' publication.

Jo, who was honest enough to tell me before it was too late that the whole thing needed a hefty rewrite, and Reagan, who drew what I wanted instead of what I asked for.

Carl, whom I have never met, but who nags me to write and Pinky, who gets things done.

Table of Contents

ONE

Why not spend two years in Canada?

Groundhog Day took the biscuit. Although I was almost calling them cookies by then. No-one believed that I'd never heard of Groundhog Day but I hadn't. Honestly. Not fond of cinemas for reasons of volume as well as finance, I hadn't even seen the film. So when a pal mentioned it in passing as a fixed reference point on the calendar, I assumed that Groundhog Day was as much a part of the 'make a fool of the daft Brit' routine as all that stuff about hunting and shooting your pumpkin for Halloween.

Groundhog Day however turned out to be real, I could tell from the fevered media build-up. It would be in a more paranoid universe than the one I inhabited that TV, radio and the *K/W Record* were all out to make a fool of me. And they were all aquiver with anticipation. So I set about an urgent piece of transatlantic research in a manner reminiscent of proper travel writers and uncovered the following – each year on February the second, an elite band of specially selected (and presumably, meteorologically prescient) groundhogs are coaxed from their hibernation burrows and encouraged to pop their heads out of doors. If their cute little noses cast shadows on the ground we're all in for six more weeks of winter. If, on the other hand, it's a bit overcast and yer actual elite weather hog doesn't see his nose's shadow, we can look forward to an early spring.

There are those who consider that this time honoured tradition has less to do with weather forecasting than with the need for a bit of a carnival by the time February comes around but I'm a convert. Especially since my first ever Groundhog Day proved so entertaining.

The movie buffs among you will have heard of Punxsutawnwy Phil of course but Ontario's favourite groundhog is – or was – Wiarton Willie. The town of Wiarton holds a Groundhog Day Festival every year. Hundreds of people turn up to see Willie predict the weather, and to sport woolly groundhog noses and ears kindly provided for them at minimal expense by local entrepreneurs.

As if all that isn't exciting enough, this year the nation was rocked by the terrible news that Willie had passed away over the winter and would therefore be making his annual prediction from beyond the grave. His demise was kept a closely guarded secret until the day itself so as not to put off the punters or spoil the festivities. And then, in a gesture of supreme poignancy, his traditional live appearance was replaced by a little furry version of lying in state. In a groundhog-sized open casket. Clutching a wistfully ceremonial carrot.

Not everyone was impressed with the dignity of the occasion. In particular, the parents of small children who had been looking forward to seeing a live sniffly cutie-pie and saw instead their first coffin, albeit a small one. Suspicions that the move may have been motivated more by concern for tourist revenue than respect for an ex-groundhog were rife.

The controversy didn't prevent a moment of silent respect during the business of Parliament or a touching eulogy from the Premier of Ontario. And good news from Pennsylvania. Punxsutawnwy Phil did not see his shadow, so – Willie or no Willie – we were in for an early spring.

The good burghers of Wiarton were hurt by all the criticism. Willie was a rare albino groundhog and his only understudy had passed on to the great meteorological lab in the sky the previous winter too. What were they supposed to do? Many people had already travelled to the festival to make a weekend of it by the time the awful truth emerged (or rather, didn't emerge) so they had reasoned that just announcing there would be no groundhog for Groundhog Day would be just as unpopular. They couldn't win. They had done their best in a crisis.

And then the really shocking news. Are you ready for this? It wasn't really Willie in the casket. It was an impostor. The brouhaha thickened. We, the concerned public, now know that Willie, when found, was in a slightly less savoury state than is commensurate with dignified lying-in-state. A stand-in was found by way of a stuffed ex-albino groundhog – one of Willie's past doppelgangers. Most shocking of all, the reason he was so touchingly arranged with a carrot on his chest was to *hide the taxidermist's label*. The nation is appalled. The papers refer to Williegate. Festival organisers are unrepentant: 'people needed to see a corpse as part of the grieving process' said a representative to the *K/W Record*. I have to say it's good to know we Brits aren't the only nation with a due regard for the dignity of our furry friends.

* * *

It started with a small ad. And the question, 'Why not?' Have you ever done that? Read an ad for some impossibly exotic job and imagined yourself blagging your way in? It's the stuff of daydreams and idle speculation, reserved for those dismal Sunday afternoons when life feels a bit grey and there are still dishes to be washed. Be careful next time you try it and beware the *why-not* moment. *Why-not* can become a serious barrier to emotional equilibrium. If you can't invent a single, solitary example of the genre it becomes impossible to think like a proper grown-up.

If I could have come up with one genuine quibble, not doing it might have been less than bare-faced cowardice. As it was, the stark choice appeared to be: apply for the opportunity of a lifetime or come to terms with the fact that you're a bit pathetic really. The dishes weren't going to make it go away either.

Let me explain. Idly scanning *The Guardian* Society Vacancies page one uneventful February morning, I happened upon a tiny ad for someone to care for an elderly lady in Canada. Live-in, full-board, two-year work visa, suit student or single parent. Well, Canada was pretty near the top of my list of places to see, I can care for elderly folk in my sleep (and often have) and if it would suit a single parent then maybe having a small but relatively house-trained youngster in tow would be an advantage for a change. Yeah, why not? Sling in job, rent out house, give away car and swan off to Canada for two years, people do it all the time.

Obviously it couldn't really be that simple. I spent an entire day mining the recesses of my imagination for hitches before even faxing a request for more details. I mentally rehearsed every excruciating detail (including fostering the cats) before taking the less than precipitous step of expressing an interest. I made lists for goodness sake. Looking for the *why-not.* But there wasn't one. It was disconcertingly feasible.

And then, all of a sudden it has been on your mind for a whole day and you have accidentally composed the letter in your sleep and well, who'd want to wonder on their deathbed what might have happened if they'd had the courage to send it?

Interest expressed, return fax read and it sounded like fun. A faintly wacky old lady who can sometimes remember liking Monty Python, regular time off and use of the car for touring. In the days before Alzheimer's took so much of this lady away she had loved to be surrounded by children so the family considered that a child in the house might be a positive benefit. There would be visas for us both and help with finding a school.

Clearly what I needed was some outside assistance with finding a *why-not* or two. Real pros and cons from real people who are not approaching a mid-life crisis. So I let the beast escape. Starting with the sort of people who were likely to be excited by the idea naturally, there was no point in running it past Mother too soon. After all the good reason not to do it would emerge sooner or later and then I wouldn't have to.

I began with someone relatively easy to convince. After a mammoth tour of Australia, Rachael knows her international hitches inside-out but was probably predisposed to egg me on. Predictably enough her considered opinion went along the lines of 'go for it'. Next, Alison, the pal I can always rely on to pour cold water on my dafter exploits from boyfriends to tattoos. Alison's verdict: 'go for it'. There was nothing for it but to call in the artillery – yes, dear reader, I finally consulted my mother. The Mumster, true to her calling as long-suffering parent of a bit of an oddball took longer to get there via probing questions, interesting angles and intelligent quibbles but ended up with words to the effect of 'go for it'.

The cold water came in the shape of a nine year old boy. Ben isn't sure if he wants to leave his friends for that long. We've looked on the map and yes, we would be able to visit the whale he adopted and he really wants to see all the mountains and lakes and stuff...but going to a strange school...suppose he doesn't make friends? I suggest we nag his school to get on-line double quick so that he can email them all with fascinating travelogues whenever he wants to. This helps a bit but not much. Which is fair enough. Is it unreasonable to need a bit of time to come round to a huge new idea when you're nine? It took me a whole day after all and I'm almost grown-up.

Was it fair to use my parental clout to persuade him? Did I really believe that he'd be bound to make friends wherever he went and would love it when he got there? Did I need to believe it at that stage? Isn't one step at a time is the way most people do things? The most important question seemed to be 'will we ever forgive ourselves for not having a go?'

And then of course, it became horribly clear that we had no choice. I'd told too many people to be allowed to back out.

* * *

I'd never applied for a job by fax before, the exotic new experiences had begun. I toddled up our road to the local newsagent's with a CV and a long letter pointing out why we were the perfect choice. I'm actually quite well qualified on paper, I'd hate you to think that seeing the world, having a bit of an adventure and wanting the word 'international' somewhere on my CV were my only motives. With ten years in the London Ambulance Service under my belt, two more caring for an elderly relative of my own and a psychology degree I probably did have the ideal credentials. The family were looking for someone who could handle the psychological challenges of Alzheimer's Disease as well as the physical effects of old age. They also wanted someone who could be lively and stimulating enough to keep their mother young rather than help her grow old, so I tried to make us sound as interesting, jolly and eccentric as possible. Not difficult if you take into account my recent foray into the world of stand-up comedy and Ben's famously unorthodox end-of-term performance from *The Jungle Book* involving a real banana.

I'd never applied for a job on the basis of off-the-wallness before either. Had I made us sound too irresponsible? Did this family really want (or need) an all-singing, all-dancing music hall act caring for their mother? Should I send a more sober PS? Or grow up and stop fretting?

In the meantime the maps were out and the imaginations ran riot. Everyone pitched in:

'Grizzly bears!'

'Polar bears!'

'Eskimos; mountains; Mounties (I liked the sound of this one); lakes; whales…'

'It doesn't look far from New York, you could go and see the Statue of Liberty, wow look it's near Niagara Falls!'

By the time the phone call from Canada came, Ben was converted and we were on the interview list. Pat, the elderly lady's daughter, will fly to England to meet the likely candidates next week. There are a few on the list but she likes the sound of us best (hooray) and yes you can see whales from the beach in the summer. She will bring videos and photos with her so that we can meet her Mum in a virtual sort of way and see our potential house and garden; the first of two Canadian homes. Sooner or later we'd all move from Mum's present house in Ontario to an island in British Columbia near to where Pat lives, in preparation for Mum's long term care. The point of the two-year carer is to cover for Pat while she builds the new house and organises the move. She appears to want us to be happy and we begin to talk as though it will be us in the end.

Meanwhile in class 4C Ben (converted by the idea of living on An Island) is holding the floor.

'Please Miss, can you get the computer on the internet because I might be going to live in Canada and I want to email about it.' Apparently one of the school's computers might be on-line soon and he is already composing his first dispatch and finding out how to spell whale. He is now so excited that if it doesn't happen I doubt I'll be forgiven.

'What did your teacher say when you told them about it Ben?'

'Everybody was very surprised. They said they'd miss me…that was a bit sad.'

'Would you be sad?'

'Only a bit.'

* * *

Uncertainty does strange things to the psyche. Before the trip to meet us, Pat had to work her way doggedly through a minefield of regulations relating to employing us rotten foreigner types. We have moved from fax to email for speed of updates, much to the disappointment of the chaps at the newsagent's. As said emails race to and fro across the Atlantic, we have veered from enthusiasm to disappointment so many times that the pair of us are now too dazed to know whether we want to go to Canada or not. First there was the difficulty with my qualifications. I have too many. Canadian Human Resources smell a rat because graduates don't do care work. Pat found a way round this by calling me an administrator, only to discover the next problem – bringing a dependant into the country. You can do this if you are a carer but not if you are an administrator. Or something. A kindly person somewhere in the government hierarchy advised her to change the job description one more time with yet another job title and hey presto, it's OK. I think I'm a Nurse Orderly now.

The email beginning 'I think I've found a loophole…' was followed by several days of silence during which I

bitterly regretted telling anyone I'd seen the wretched ad
in the first place and made a mental note to eschew *The
Guardian* henceforth. Well, on Wednesdays anyway. By the
time the email beginning 'I'll be in England tomorrow...'
arrived we were too wrung out with waiting for it to get
excited.

Then we met. Pat and I had long lists of practical and
incisive questions carefully prepared in order to make best
use of the short time she had available. Time spent grinning
inanely at each other, saying things like 'I suppose I should,
ask you some questions' and dissolving into laughter instead.
Neither of us quite knew what was expected and it showed
but giggling seemed promising enough at the time. We have
seen photos of the house, garden and school, and a video
of Pat's Mum pottering happily about in her kitchen. In all
the excitement it's easy to forget that she is the one whose
comfort and peace of mind matter the most. Pat thinks she'll
like us but who can tell? We have given her some photos of
us to take home with her so that she can stick them up on
the kitchen wall with name labels attached. All the current
respite carers are on the kitchen wall with name labels,
so the plan is that by the time we get there we will be no
more or less familiar than all the other ever-changing, half-
remembered faces who drift in and out of view.

As for the photos she's given us, well, everything looks
big and alien and odd. We now know that the nearest school
is ten minutes walk away, there's a wood at the bottom of
the street and Niagara Falls is about two hours away. The
whales will have to wait for the move to British Columbia.
And we really are going to do this.

Eventually the giggling subsided and we managed to
discuss businesslike things such as domestic, financial and
travel arrangements. The lists were dusted off – who pays
for the flight, when are we needed, who does the shopping,
pays for the petrol? Then with the initial lists scribbled over,

a new one began. Things To Do Next. It doesn't include panicking, maybe it should? Although presumably I'll require no reminding if and when it becomes appropriate.

Top of the new list is the final hurdle, Canadian Immigration. Who are not the same as Canadian Human Resources, that was just Round One. Pat's fight. The next battle is mine. There are forms to be submitted in person, more forms to be posted, letters to collect, photos to take, interviews to arrange. Only once we have been 'processed' will they decide whether or not I am the sort of person who deserves a visa, so it seems a good idea to stay numb rather than excited for a little longer.

A bizarre addition to the pile of paperwork is a fax Pat has received from Channel 4 TV. They would like to cover our story for part of their *Moving People* series. They are planning a season on people moving from one country to another instead of just from house to house. On a foraging expedition through the nation's job pages in search of likely émigrés they spotted the same ad that I did. Would Pat please ask whoever she recruits if they'd be interested in having a camera follow their every move? She did. Would we? I'm not sure. Thinking about it is next on the list.

* * *

The Canadian High Commission is open to visitors from eight until eleven each weekday morning. We arrived at ten to nine on a Monday and joined a very long queue. Not to apply for our visas you understand, just to check out what to do with all the pieces of paper. Fortunately I'd packed a vast picnic to keep Ben amused during the wait. Unfortunately there were signs everywhere asking us politely in English and French not to consume our *nourissement* on the premises. Oh yes, they speak French in bits of Canada don't they?

The nice man explained all the pieces of paper, gave me a detailed list of all the additional bits of paper they required (good grief it's a thesis) and cheered me greatly by mentioning that once I'd completed the paper chase I could come back and make the application in person if I was in a hurry, then we could have a decision the same day. This was indeed great news as it meant that, with a little hustling for the relevant letters, we would know before Pat flew back to Canada whether or not we would be allowed to join her. Pat and I hustled. By the end of Tuesday we were sorted. We wrote letters from her to me, letters from me to her and hastily put them together with letters to and from the Canadian Employment Bureau. All my certificates and references had to be copied and labelled, forms filled in duplicate, a solicitor's letter or two, then Ben and I had a mad ten minutes in the photo booth and we were ready to hit the Consulate again first thing Wednesday morning.

I decided to get there a bit earlier to cut down on waiting time so we arrived at twenty past eight and joined an even longer queue. This time it was the first of many. We queued to tell the receptionist what we wanted, we queued to pay our landing fees – discovering in passing that they were non-refundable – we then queued to be 'seen'. Waiting, sweaty-palmed for the final interview I rehearsed all the possible objections there might be to me caring for a Canadian senior person. Mentally fielding each with earnest insight and as much psychobabble as one can glean in a whole hour or two of taking an interest in Alzheimer's research, I felt more and more like an illegal immigrant as each minute passed. When they finally called our names I jumped like a frightened rabbit caught in the headlights of an approaching juggernaut.

The interview went relatively well after I had rearranged all the papers that shot off my lap at juggernaut time. An official smiled at us, asked a couple of token questions, wished us luck and the juggernaut trundled off into the distance. It would revisit me occasionally but I didn't know that then.

* * *

You think I've got my visa now don't you? Nobody had yet mentioned medicals, they keep that up their sleeves until you think you're on your way. Before we finally get the magic pieces of paper in our hands Ben and I have to be prodded, listened to, x-rayed and wee-tested. And of course there's another fee (non-refundable). Then the doctor sends the results to Canada House by carrier pigeon. Then we get our visa. I'm fairly certain we don't present any significant risk to the health of the Canadian nation but it's one more way of putting off any real celebration. You wouldn't believe how tiring it is being Nearly Excited.

In an effort to postpone any irrevocable planning a little longer I telephoned the researcher from *Moving People* to tell her I didn't approve of reality TV. Then I started to tell the story. They have a way of seeming interested that sneaks round your defences don't they? I know this but I quite enjoyed telling the story anyway. Reliving how fast everything seemed to have fallen into place reminded me why I'm currently up to my ears in bits of paper and exhausted from near-excitement. Maybe a good way to survive the frustration would be to see the whole shooting match through someone else's eyes.

They would like to send someone along to do a sort of screen test. If they decide to use our story they would want to film the packing, the leaving party, our last night at home and the sad farewells at the airport. They would then come and visit us at the other end for an update. Pat has agreed to this bit, she wants the world to know more about Alzheimer's and has already given permission for them to film her Mum. Ben fancies being on telly. I've swallowed my cultural arrogance and tentatively agreed, although I'd like to make it clear right now that I'm only a little flattered by the attention.

They'll be out of luck with the sad farewells though. I've already decided to slope off quietly when the time comes, refuse all offers of lifts to the airport and avoid the tearful hanky brigade completely. I don't want Ben to spend the entire flight thinking about who he's leaving behind, it might feel less like a jolly jape. I suppose there ought to be a party though. Now I come to think of it there has to be a party. Perhaps I'll compromise and have a party.

* * *

Off for the medicals today. The doctor said 'where are the rest of the forms?' in his best bedside manner voice. Back to the Consulate first thing Monday morning.

TWO

Of course I'm emigrating you know

My slippers were soggy with dew and my nightshirt danced up and down under my coat as I moved, relatively stealthily, across the lawn. Not that I cared how I looked. It was dawn and I was on a mission. Half way across Steffi's front garden I spied my quarry and pounced, the dandelion was mine. Big, fat and juicy. Safely back in Zuscha's kitchen I gave it an admiring glance before consigning it, a tad guiltily, to the dustbin. A moment of pride. My quick thinking had averted a crisis.

'How's the new job going Carolyn?'

'Great thanks, I stole a dandelion today.'

Life had become very strange. Why did I do it? Because the *why-nots*, when they happened were too few. And by then I was on the juggernaut anyway.

* * *

They are real now though, the *why-nots*. The first, as I realise that emigrating is surprisingly expensive. Students may head off into the unknown with a toothbrush, a pair of knickers and 50p in change to bribe a border guard; but middle aged ladies with dependants don't get away so lightly. It started with the cost of the pointless private medical with some retired buffoon in Harley Street who clearly has friends in embassies. What he told them that a note from my GP wouldn't have covered I'm not quite sure but one doesn't argue with the people who have one's reputation as an intrepid explorer at stake.

Incidentally, since neither of us has TB, diabetes or syphilis the visa looks certain enough to risk a little forward planning. Provisional date of departure, April the third; provisional cost of travel insurance, luggage, clothing for extremes of temperature, camera repairs and renovation of tumble-down house to renting-out standard – 'Ben we need to do a boot sale.'

It seemed like a good idea at the time. Turn out all the things we won't be needing, don't have room to store, or that Ben doesn't play with any more, pop them into the car and turn them into cash. I had never attempted, or even attended a boot sale before, probably something to do with enjoying listening to *The Archers Omnibus* on a Sunday morning. In the warm.

I can now state without any fear of inaccuracy that I will never attend, let alone attempt one again. There is an art to this business that I absolutely can't fathom, everyone else seems to know exactly what your bits and bobs are worth but they aren't going to tell you. It's clearly more fun to be scathingly amused by the ignorant novice. Within five minutes of setting up our stall I regressed to being the little girl who didn't know how to play rounders. Nobody explained the rules then either and it was just as hard not to cry. Having risen at dawn, carried an entire car full of boxes down the stairs, unloaded them all at the other end and missed the episode after John's accident into the bargain, I was in no mood to have my entire life picked over and sniffed at. 'You won't get a pound for that luv.'

But I digress. Emigrating is also remarkably tiring. We are presently half way through March. If I am going to have turned out, sorted, stored and packed away all our worldly goods, spring-cleaned and repaired the house, selected lodgers, earned enough to pay for it all and finished icing all outstanding cakes orders by the third of April I'm going to be seriously short of sleep.

Here we go digressing again. Carolyn's Cakes may possibly be irrelevant to most of the rest of the adventure but deserve a mention anyway because of The Wedding, which has complicated the planning somewhat. The cake decorating has been an enjoyable and lucrative little sideline for many years but is becoming a bit of a headache just now, everyone wants 'one more before you go'. Concentrating on the finer points of one's sugar *bas relief* isn't easy when your mind is on ringing the bank and the tax man to tell them you're leaving the country. I have started politely to decline new orders but The Wedding Cake can't be avoided. Said wedding is planned for June, the bride is a friend and I'd already pocketed a generous deposit before answering Pat's ad. After a complicated phone call or two I have come up with a master plan for almost being in two places at once. It goes like this:

1) Make three hexagonal rich fruit cakes before I go.
2) Entrust cakes and brandy bottle to bride-to-be who will religiously dose and turn cakes (and possibly self) once a month.
3) Note down where I stash the box of nozzles/cutters/patterns etc.
4) Try not to lose note.

5) Fly back for two weeks' holiday in June, agreed with Pat at interview. The 'rota' she has proposed for me involves a pattern of two months working 24/7 followed by two weeks off so this will naturally fall in my first patch of planned holiday.

6) Unearth box of tricks.

7) Marzipan, ice and decorate to perfection as ever, construct terrifyingly lifelike sugar orchids and generally behave as though I am still North London's answer to Jane Asher.

8) Go to wedding and gloat about being a globetrotting sugar artiste.

9) Return to Canada exhausted.

What do you mean? Of course it will work.

* * *

Meanwhile there is definite progress on the organisation front. Friend-of-a-friend has offered the cats a new home, Rachael is going to foster my pictures that are too big to fit under the stairs and the monster Swiss Cheese Plant and Mum will adopt my mobile phone. Well, when I say that Rachael will foster my pictures I am being a little disingenuous. She is merely reclaiming pictures that were too big to go under her stairs when she packed her home into a cupboard and headed off to the Antipodes a few years ago. I very kindly offered to foster one or two of my faves from her art school past while she was away. When she returned I went all wheedley and pathetic about how much I'd miss them and how wonderful they looked on my walls and managed thus to kidnap them for several years. They are probably no longer mine.

I had a wistful sort of moment in Sainsbury's while returning to the shelves a trolley-full of cat food loaded under automatic pilot. Not buying cat food was the first real change in routine. It was so poignant I had to cheer myself up by playing with our smart new suitcases. Super-duper posh ones, with wheels. Never had wheels before – the cases, not us – I smile at them from time to time by way of a break from the spring cleaning. Proper travellers have luggage with wheels don't they?

Ben is making significant progress too. Not only has he added curling and fishing to his list of things to learn to do in Canada but his research has unearthed the stupendous news that Canada has slugs the size of bananas. Called, oddly enough, Banana Slugs. He's therefore about halfway through packing away his very best stones.

* * *

The camera from *Moving People* finally arrived for an experimental day's filming, to see if we 'worked as a story'. Naturally I will now be a little disappointed if we don't, having realised that viewing the hard work part of packing up a three bedroom house in under a month through someone else's eyes just might make be the only thing that makes it tolerable. Although I may have blown it with my usual approach to conversation, i.e. say the first thing than comes into your head regardless of context. 'What will you miss while you're away?' might have been meant to generate something more thought provoking than 'just *The Archers* I think' but I was still smarting from a disappointing phone call to the BBC. No it isn't broadcast on the World Service.

Happily the party needs no further pondering. Ben and I have decided to hold a multi-generation effort on our last Sunday here. We have been printing and distributing invitations in industrial quantities, mainly in order to avoid sorting out, emptying and cleaning the cupboard under the stairs ready to receive Stuff. I've been doing a lot of avoiding the cupboard under the stairs. Who wouldn't? And don't tell me that the cupboard under your stairs is squeaky clean and stacked neatly because I won't believe you. The most recent errand to suddenly become urgent was the taking of my camera back to Dixon's to complain about a recalcitrant flashgun. 'I'm leaving the country shortly' I announced somewhat sniffily 'and I must have a fully functional camera'. It turned out that I had inadvertently moved some button or other and that the camera is as fully functional as a camera can get. Being under the stairs suddenly seemed like a relatively attractive option.

I've been announcing my plans to total strangers alarmingly often. I have this urge to say 'of course I'm emigrating you know' to all and sundry, rather in the manner of someone who is terribly sprightly for their age. Most people are relatively tolerant, after the initial startled-and-faintly-hunted look that goes with realising that it's your turn to cop today's nutter.

Ben is devising a farewell performance for the end of term talent show at school. There will be a display of magic tricks to surpass all previous entertainments. I think I can safely reveal that the emphasis will be on disappearing hankies but beyond this my lips are sealed. He has also finished packing away his stones ready for storage. Packed carefully with them are his experiments, at least the ones that haven't gone slimy and smelly (yet). I wonder exactly what we'll unearth in two years' time but am sufficiently impressed that he is contributing real work to allow a little autonomy.

Ben's progress is countered by a bit of a hitch on the feline front. The cats are still with us. The family who thought they'd like them have changed their minds so they are back at the top of my 'things to worry about' list, along with finding takers for our pushbikes and Ben's cabin bed. I have also had to go out and buy a trolley load of cat food.

And what's more, I am down with a horrible gooey cold. Nothing as dramatic as flu but one of those really drippy, shivery, wobbly-when-you-stand-up sorts of colds. Since the threshold of a new life is an inconvenient time to be ill I decided to pamper myself, cancel some work and rest a lot. While resting I found time to wonder whether presenting myself back at Canada House and looking desperate might hurry the visa up a bit. There had been no news since I sent in the medical results (maybe I'd been right about the carrier pigeon) the pre-Easter flights were filling up fast and Pat, back in Canada and in urgent need of a carer, was starting to fret about delays and overbooked flights. I dragged myself and a large box of tissues onto the underground, infecting the travelling public with reckless abandon. 'Oh well' they said when I got there, 'we may as well do it today then'.

Yes, I now have the magic pieces of paper in my hand, the flight is booked for Good Friday – just a week late – and I can only wonder how much longer it might have taken if I hadn't gone down with a cold.

* * *

The cold-induced irreversible steps are under way. I've spent a day on the telephone cancelling bank accounts, redirecting tax returns and arranging to cut off the phone. I have handed in my notice. I don't have any regrets (yet) or many doubts (yet) but turning down work definitely has the faint whiff of burning boats about it. I won't mention the juggernaut again here, a certain level of metaphor mixing ought to be allowable in my heightened state of anxiety but even I can see that would be over the top.

I'm also getting very sentimental about my friends. People keep ringing to arrange to see us 'before you go'. We've been treated to lunches and suppers, meals in, meals out, cards have arrived and little prezzies. I'm particularly charmed by our lucky travelling socks, which we will definitely be wearing for the flight. And joys of joys, the kindest family in the whole of Wiltshire has volunteered to send regular tape cassettes of *The Archers*. The party has snowballed into something enormous and Ben and I keep telling each other how lucky we are to have such nice people in our lives. Although it is always possible they're just glad to see the back of us.

The hard labour is coming along well. You should see the cupboard under my stairs! The wedding cakes are baked, Ben's bed has a new home as do the bikes. The bookshelves are empty and the kitchen cupboards sparkly clean. The house is fit to advertise, the rooms are fit to rent.

The cats may finally have found a home. Friend of another friend is popping over to interview them next week. Am hoping they will behave and be suitably cute. Must remember to tell Ben to keep quiet about Pickle's fondness for weeing on his beanbag and Lilly's habit of dancing on the ansaphone until it talks to her and clears itself of unheard messages. Getting them both into a box on the same day will be a challenge but no doubt it will amuse the cameras. Yes, Channel 4 have been back in touch. We are now an officially interesting story, Ben is declared a 'natural' and they have decided to film the school talent show too.

This ought to be great news. Sadly we are in the throes of recovering from a totally terrible dress rehearsal. Everything that could possibly go wrong did and now some of his friends think they know how the magic is done. Needless to say this is devastating and the prospect of a TV camera on the big day isn't helping. Neither am I, nothing I can say is any reassurance at all, I've tried 'bad rehearsals are traditional'. I've also tried 'your friends are just jealous' and 'hey, we could always leave the country'. But none of it is wise, true or even funny just now. Thank goodness the Banana Slugs are only two weeks away.

* * *

Emotional journey Stage 4, Irritated. (For those of you taking notes: Stage 1, Nearly Excited; Stage 2, Anxious;

Stage 3, Sentimental.) It began at the party. On the surface it ranked as one of my better dos. Lots of people drifting in and out, proving themselves capable of eating, drinking and talking to each other without much assistance from me. Our tame producer from Channel 4 arrived with a camera and a bottle – a touch I found very endearing. Her name is Laura and she will be following us around right through to Canada now. Friends old and new were telling each other how wonderful/brave/funny/insert-compliment-here we were and how much they would miss us, it ought to have been lovely.

Conversely by the time the tearful farewells began I couldn't be bothered with anyone and wanted them all to go away with the minimum of fuss. Where did that come from? I seem to have put all the things I should be feeling about my loved ones in a box and nailed the lid down tight. I don't actually want to hear that we'll be missed, even if it's just politeness. All of a sudden I am crabby and have had to make an executive decision to duck out of all other farewell efforts in case I say something I'll regret. Otherwise we'll have no friends left to come home to.

Or to commiserate with if we don't go after all. There has been a slight crisis over the flight. Pat booked the tickets for us from over there with a Canadian charter airline that doesn't have offices here. We are supposed to collect the tickets from Stansted Airport on the day we leave. In efficiency mode, and having run out of utilities (and total strangers) to inform of our plans, I rang Stansted to ask who we should contact for up-to-date information, delays and suchlike. Their response to my enquiry ran along the lines of 'No flights to Canada until May dear. No it's not on my computer, shall I put you on to Gatwick?... Gatwick charters go to Toronto...Are you sure it's not Gatwick... Shall I transfer you anyway?...Are you sure...'

Carolyn Steele

It was the middle of the night in Canada so I wore a hole in the carpet waiting for a reasonable hour to wake Pat for a mutual panic. The Toronto office assured her the flight existed. Stansted reassured me it didn't and made increasingly desperate attempts to fob me off with a switchboard operator at Gatwick. Solving the mystery took most of the day. The flight exists all right but it isn't in anyone's computer because it's the first of the season so there's no rep in the UK yet to have a computer to put it in. Suddenly the idea of picking up tickets from the airport felt a tad risky, if they can lose a whole flight my tickets don't stand a chance. After spending a fortune on transatlantic phone calls to try and track down a place I might be able to collecting them from, I ferreted out a travel agent in Kensington who has dealings with the relevant airline. I haven't started seeing the world yet but I'm certainly getting around some of the finer parts of London. Kensington here I come, it would be nice to sleep again before we leave.

I have been losing sleep over a lot lately. The talent show for example. After the totally terrible rehearsal, we worked hard on fall-back measures to cover for technical hitches on the day. Ben bounced back eventually and woke on the last day of term supremely confident. I of course approached the occasion with all the signs and symptoms of major trauma. You know though, don't you, that the entire performance went without a hitch. Producing a pound coin from the headmaster's ear went down particularly well, as did the final baffling appearance of sweeties. And I am left drained and beaten into a pulp by my inability to choose the right things to worry about. Why stress about emigrating when you can be a shivering heap over an end-of-term school show? It makes so much more sense. After a good cry I felt a lot better and we can't wait to see it on TV now. Although I have my doubts about the bit where, seeing the

24

state I was in Laura pointed the camera at me with a wicked grin, 'so, how are you feeling Mum?'

The house is almost empty. My packing and squirreling away of things we aren't taking with us has been so efficient that I keep having to root around and find things we still need that were stashed away weeks ago. Like shoes. I placed a suitcase full of the sort of clothes and shoes no-one wears for comfort in the loft, ready to reappear when I return and need to look smart again. If I ever get another job after it's all over that is. It dawned on me at one o'clock in the morning, after a glass of wine too many, that my work shoes were packed with them despite one final shift the following morning. Now I only have two fears in life but one of them happens to be the climbing of ladders. (Slugs, the other. I may have a spot of trouble with the monster Canadian version.) After negotiating a stepladder in the dark whilst tired and emotional to retrieve a pair of shoes packed in haste, I refused to put anything else away anywhere in case I needed it again before we left. Now I'm running out of time. I'll never get the rest done by Friday.

THREE

I can't say Jell-O

So what would you do with your last night at home? The boxes are stowed, the cases are packed and you can't deal with toothbrushes until the morning because if you pack them you will have to unpack them again to clean your teeth with. It ought to be sort of momentous but it's hard to do momentous on your own and you appear to have accidentally rejected all your friends, no doubt for reasons that made sense at the time. Getting drunk is probably a daft idea getting-up-in-the-morning-wise and just watching TV like you normally do seems inappropriately pedestrian. What do you do? You sit and think. And then you get frightened.

What have I done to us? I'm dragging my son into the unknown to live somewhere we've never seen, with people we've never met. I'm expecting him to be happy and take it all in his stride without the slightest idea what it'll be like. I should be dobbing myself in to the NSPCC, not swanning around in front of TV cameras pretending to be intrepid. I am an idiot. And I am lonely for both of us.

Our worldly goods are crammed into two suitcases (with wheels), the regulation two pieces of hand luggage and a Shawn the Sheep backpack full of games for the journey, which we're planning to call a handbag. Everything else has been jettisoned because two months ago I thought we were both so clever and mature and original that we could take ourselves anywhere and handle anything. I do know that the hangover will be a significant disadvantage in the morning but I think there are some odds and ends of unidentified bottles in an easily accessible box. Besides, I ought to check under the stairs one more time. Here's to the idiot. Cheers.

* * *

The hangover might have presented more of a problem if I'd needed to drive us to Canada but as luck would have it we were flying. Even better, one of my wiser decisions had involved accepting a lift to the airport. Despite my protestations on the vexed subject of hanky-waving a particularly insistent pal had managed to convince me that an extra pair of hands with the luggage wouldn't be too distressing. That ride turned out to be the best leaving present of all, I got away with not focusing for an hour or two in the morning and, joy of joys, we didn't have to pack it.

I like airports, all those people going somewhere, we're not foolhardy here, just two more travellers – one large, one small. A child can be a useful piece of travelling equipment at times, far handier than those inflatable pillowy things with a seam that digs into your neck however you try to snuggle into it. Hard-bitten customs officials get the urge to bleat at a jogging Shawn the Sheep backpack full of toys; cabin staff find it in their hearts to try and laugh when the little chap reinvents the joke and puts the sweet in his ear. Ben beat me at every game unearthed from Shawn on the way, including chess, much to the amusement of our fellow passengers. In my defence I have to admit that I've always been appalling at chess but I didn't even win at Pass the Pigs; a truly inspired travelling gift by the way. A game that not only fits in your pocket but inspires conversations of such bizarre silliness as to generate instant friends in airport lounges. Next time you are required to wish someone bon voyage, be sure to say it with pigs.

Laura was due to meet us at Toronto airport to film the great arrival. She was looking forward to catching us exhausted, jet lagged and struggling with our cases. To this end she had taken an earlier flight from Heathrow, intending to be all set up and ready for us by the time we'd cleared Immigration. Which we did with relative ease, oddly enough. I was expecting plenty more grilling and shuffling of papers and all manner of pointless red tape, possibly involving carrier pigeons, but the chap took Ben on a tour of the cells they put deportees in instead. Don't pack a pillow, pack a child.

I don't know quite why neither Channel 4 nor I thought to enquire as to the number of terminals at Pearson International, Toronto. Perhaps we all though of it as just not very international but scheduled flights and charters don't mix, so while Laura spent an hour or so at Terminal Three searching for a lost microphone case, we spent an hour or so at Terminal One searching for her. After having her paged several times and delaying our ground transportation (that's a bus to you) twice, we gave in to overwhelming exhaustion and allowed ourselves to be whisked away to the twin cities of Kitchener/Waterloo, Ontario, to begin our new little lives, assuming she'd catch up with us sooner or later. (Which she did but we were so used to being tailed by then that we almost didn't notice. Sorry Laura.)

This crisis at the airport provided our first taste of culture shock. Everybody helped us. Not a jobsworth in sight, no-one from the 'if it isn't on the shelf we haven't got it' school of customer service, just polite co-operation with a cheerful smile, a 'you're welcome' and the distinct impression that somebody cares. You want to page a daft message to Terminal Three again? 'Certainly Ma'am, right away.' 'Oh you're very welcome.' You want to rearrange the bus driver's schedule again? 'No problem Ma'am, when would you like to leave?' 'You're welcome.' I thought they were being sarcastic for a while but that can't be it because everyone is the same. Not just in the shops and eateries where presumably they are paid to be pleasant but everybody, everywhere.

All Canadians appear to say 'you're welcome' all the time. That takes a bit of getting used to. I was taught to say it as a toddler of course but I seem to recall that only toddlers still say 'you're welcome' to people back in London. Which predisposes me to be charmed by all and sundry, since even a six-foot square, bear-shaped and impossibly moustachioed Canadian policeman sounds faintly like a toddler to me when he's saying 'you're welcome Ma'am.'

As national sayings go, it is almost as popular as the true Canadian fave 'how are you?' Everyone wants to know how I am today. It's a lot more disconcerting than 'have a nice day', especially when it sounds relatively genuine, as there is the perennial uncertainly as to whether the enquirer ought to expect an answer. Is it like 'How do you do?' Do you just say it back or should one construct a reply? There seems to be a bit of a competition in shops and banks etc. to see who can get it in first. I am beginning to wonder if wages are docked when the customer wins. It'll be a long time before this one manages it though, I have twigged that some sort of reply is appropriate but I'm still tussling with the most appropriate version, 'Well the jet lag is wearing off nicely now thank you but I'm still a bit confused by people keep asking me how I am all the time.' Or possibly 'fine thanks, how are you?' Or maybe 'well, I'm feeling terrible since you ask, I've got this pain…'

You don't have to know anyone to get a wave and a howarya, just being sentient is enough to make you worth the time of day. *Due South* is real, these are the politest, friendliest people on earth and that's before they hear the accent. Once we're established as English, we may as well be royalty. I have the feeling that everyone in Canada wants us to feel at home and I wish we did. If only to make all the nice people happy.

* * *

What was I expecting? I didn't know until the surprises started. It now appears that I was expecting trees and space and stuff, so although there are indeed huge expanses of trees plus plenty of the aforementioned space, they aren't too alarming. I wasn't expecting the sort of trivial, everyday oddities that I've only ever seen before in films. Fire hydrants for example. And mail boxes. Now they are seriously weird. Where are Tom and Jerry, Top Cat and the other characters who inhabit exotic places with such bizarre street furniture? I am walking through a film set and they are probably round the corner. Vertical exhaust pipes on lorries – where is the Road Runner? Will I bump into Clint Eastwood shortly?

I know it's a cliché but the small things catch you out. It's all very well memorising the exchange rate to work out what everything costs but it's embarrassing to have to ask a stranger to identify a quarter in your small change so that you can use a public telephone. And how on earth can one behave like a citizen of the world when the shop assistant wants to know if one has a dime? It's bad enough that the five and ten cent coins are the wrong sizes, being expected to cope with nicknames is just plain unreasonable. I would probably be OK somewhere a bit more touristy but this is small-town Canada where people just live and work, they are not used to foreigners handing over a fistful of change and asking them to take whatever they need.

At least I know now what the chap at the airport meant when he said 'you'll need a Loonie for the cart Ma'am.' At the time I just smiled pleasantly, pretended not to speak English and struggled with my luggage, wondering vaguely if it was some sort of job creation scheme. I am now proud to be able to report that a Loonie is a dollar coin. There's a Loon on the back you see. A Loon is a type of duck. Which is why the two-dollar coin is a Twoonie. Or something. And what's more, while I'm moaning about money, writing cheques is sheer hell. I was a fully functioning adult a week ago but they write the date backwards here and my self-respect is crumbling.

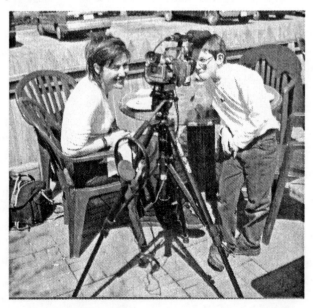

Laura and her camera caught up with us in the end

If it's not money upsetting the equilibrium it's language. We're out of cartoons now and into songs. How can you possibly say things like *sidewalk* and *downtown* in an English accent without sounding as though you are auditioning for a Broadway musical? I can just about say *drugstore* without feeling silly but *Jell-O* is a complete non-starter. I'll have to utter it sooner or later of course, because jelly is jam. And what's more, crisps are chips. Ben and I have resorted to pointing. Which would be less degrading if we were learning a new language.

Eating out is an exercise in multiple-choice exam technique. There's no such thing as a cup of coffee. It is long or short, double or single, latte or espresso or possibly Americano and what flavour beans would you like? English coffee may be dishwater but at least you don't have to think before you get one. Yes I know Starbucks has introduced us Brits to the concept of complicated coffee but I'm talking downmarket caffs here, not showcases for beautiful people with tanned legs and pseudo-transatlantic attitude.

On the upside, I am definitely getting the hang of the shops. Post offices lurk in the back of drugstores (why is that do you suppose?) and there are hundreds of varieties of most things but strange little black holes where staple items ought to be.

Take pickles for example, an entire aisle devoted to pickled cucumbers but no onions. And crisps; more flavours than you can shake a stick at (including pickled cucumber) but an absence of cheese and onion. What do cucumbers have that onions don't? And why doesn't talc exist? How can a whole continent of people not use talc? Strange to think that talcum powder will be at the top of my Christmas present list this year, I usually have the stuff coming out of my ears during the festive season.

The grocery stores (not shops, workshops appear to be shops) are packed with ready meals but it's not easy to find individual ingredients, especially if you don't know what to call them or what kind of packaging to look out for. I sussed cornstarch fairly early on and am well and truly on top of the 'bag of milk' situation, although it was perturbing to start with. Now that I know they sell milk in plastic bags I can go and ask for some without a panic attack. Mince is more worrying. Why do they call it hamburger? And what should I call a hamburger? And why doesn't anyone know what I am talking about? I'm not the one with the accent.

I'll tell you another thing. There's a good few silly questions an unwary Brit can utter, instantly giving themselves away as the new kid in town. Like 'Can you park there?' I am learning not to ask, although occasionally it's fun to remind myself just how incredulous a face can become whilst still remaining polite. The concept of inadequate parking space is totally redundant in a land full of elbow-room and the sort of nonsense only a daft Londoner would come out with. (That's London, England of course. There's another quite nearby. Ben and I are planning a trip to London, Ontario shortly to buy some postcards to send home.)

Another dead giveaway; 'how big is a small one?' Nothing is small. Regular is the smallest anything gets and is usually sufficient for two.

Watching TV (I've learned not to call it telly) helps a bit and is my main source of cross-cultural education. I am glued to adverts and the local news for vocabulary hints and tips. Today's little lesson; police identikit descriptions include the category 'pot-bellied'. So much more evocative than our own 'heavily-built'. They also specify which way round wanted desperados choose to wear their baseball caps.

Some things do remain the same the world over though and after intensive research I am glad be able to report that politicians, pot-bellied or not, appear to be pretty consistent on both sides of the Atlantic. The news is full of apologies just now from the Premier of Ontario for an unwise comment regarding pregnant women spending their nutrition allowance on beer. Huge outcry, sincere apology and suddenly I feel at home again. I wonder what this guy thinks about single parents. He, Mike Harris for those of you who like facts in your travel writing, seems to produce a gaffe per year on average. The news bulletins gleefully re-run previous howlers by way of illustration. I am particularly fond of his speech about how Canadian society wouldn't have fallen apart if mothers cooked their children hot breakfasts instead of skiving off to work all the time.

* * *

All these observations are merely diverting however, a whimsical extension of being on holiday. Learning to live in someone else's house, by someone else's rules and in someone else's normality is a little tougher. I didn't know I was set in my ways until I inherited new ones. I'd like to be able to listen to the radio in the morning, to turn off the TV when no-one is watching it and to shoo cats off the kitchen table. I'd like to be able to keep out of the sun when it's hot. And open a window when a cool breeze blows. But most of all I'd like to be able to tidy up.

I wasn't aware of being clean and tidy until we moved here. In fact, I wasn't clean and tidy until we moved here. I've always thought of myself as a tad slovenly in the housework department to be honest but our new home makes me twitch with the kind of repressed urge to get the marigolds on that you generally associate with mothers-in-law. It's almost the next *why-not*.

Pat's Mum empties the contents of cupboards and drawers all over the house by way of nocturnal entertainment. She also collects stones and pebbles from the garden and roots up small plants to be brought home as special prizes. The kitchen table acts as holding-pen for most of these outdoor goodies, where they mingle with forgotten treasures from the previous night's scavenging, a selection of partly finished jigsaw puzzles and a lost half-a-meal or two. If the kitchen table is overflowing the sink provides an effective backup, with or without dishes in, and if the sink is too full of muddy roots to accept more, anywhere else in the house will do at a pinch. There is little point in trying to put anything away; the cupboards and drawers will be re-emptied again each night and the garden re-uprooted every day. Over the months Pat has given up the struggle. With constant vigilance it's almost possible to keep small corners of Ben's room and mine mud-free – although we both get the occasional gift of a little pile of grimy pebbles left affectionately on the end of the bed – but the rest of the house lays beneath a permanent coating of rocks, roots, wilted greenery, more pebbles, bits of jigsaw puzzle and… stuff, in a layer reminiscent of the day Ben opened a packet of Rice Krispies all on his own. Only muddier.

Her name is Adrienne but we are to call her Zuscha. She will be my job and my life from here on in and I will be her shadow. Adrienne may be her name but the only people who use it are the ones who don't matter, insignificant official people and nosy locals, it's a dead giveaway and generates instant non-cooperation. Zuscha is Dutch for 'little sister', a pet name that has signified family affection down the years. It seems to bypass the confusion a little so we all use it.

Alzheimer's-type dementia isn't Zuscha's only challenge, she is also somewhat deaf so all conversations are conducted at maximum volume. To complicate matters further she has diabetes, combined with the inevitable sweet tooth. I hadn't known about the diabetes when we left England. It was Easter wasn't it? The Bunny had thoughtfully secreted a few Easter eggs in our luggage so that Ben wouldn't be chocolateless when we landed. That

Bunny had to be pretty inventive, I can tell you, to ensure that Ben found his eggs and Zuscha didn't, especially as she had all night in which to work relatively unsupervised. I'd thought at packing time, whilst pretending to have forgotten that Easter was looming, that the subterfuge had been a bit complicated. Little did I know that the dissembling and cheating had only just begun.

I am developing several extra eyes and a seriously devious nature, just in time to learn the tricks of the trade with regard to shopping. Every confectionary counter we pass poses a potential chocolate standoff hazard but fortunately Zuscha's short-term memory is poor enough for some base trickery. It cheers her up momentarily to choose some, we chat happily about the nicest brand and place it proudly in our basket, then a well thought-out distraction makes it possible to replace the contraband back on the shelf about an aisle and a half after she has picked it up. This way we enjoy our shopping trips and don't fall out over who is in charge. Or end up in hospital with a coma looming. We leave a trail of muddled goods in our wake but no-one seems to mind.

I am also starting to unravel how she inhabits her little obsessions and which ones serve her at different times of day. After dark she opens and closes curtains, locks doors and windows and checks to see who is in each of the bedrooms. In the daytime she pulls up weeds from the garden, snaffles flowers and roots from around the neighbourhood when no-one is looking and collects pocketfuls of stones and pebbles when they are. In the evening she picks up tiny bits of fluff from the carpets and when she is up and about overnight she turns out the cupboards and drawers. Usually clothes, although on an extra restless night it tends to be the cutlery drawer. Clothes are quieter. There is a sort of routine.

Most of her habits make sense if you overlay the memory loss onto a lifetime as housewife and mother. I do them myself (with the possible exception of weeding). If you close the curtains at night and open them in the morning, you are running a household. If you keep forgetting you've done it but remember that you're supposed to, you are a batty old lady. What used to be a passion for raising plants is now a tendency to rip green stuff out of every flower bed in the district. A lifelong interest in archaeology has become the precious heaps of stones and pebbles lovingly sorted on the kitchen table.

In a bid to empathise, we have taken to musing on the subject of which obsessions we are likely to carry into our own old age. I think I will probably steal cars quite a lot. When Ben takes my wheels away to keep the streets safer for other road users it will be an appalling injustice and I am sure I will just go out and find myself some more. Driving defines me, just as gardening, rock collecting and looking after people have defined Zuscha down the years. Ben thinks he may be another pebble-collector and we think we may be a step closer to Zuscha's world.

She is good humoured, good fun, devastatingly sarcastic and impossibly stubborn. Her worst excesses are saved up for those patronising souls who insist on asking her if she knows who they are. I like her. Liking isn't quite enough for the best of honest and authentic caring though, there needs to be a bit of genuine respect in the mix too and I am glad to be able to report that Zuscha is even easier to respect than she is to like.

Pat doesn't share much, it seems that Zuscha may not have said a great deal about her reasons for heading to Canada but history can fill some of the gaps. Zuscha was born in Holland, she lived through the Nazi occupation. Many of her friends were Jews and most owe their lives to her. She spent her war years working with the Dutch resistance and not just for friends, when she wasn't hiding people in her home she was smuggling babies across borders. There are hair-raising stories of her seducing Nazi officers to distract their attention from the human contents of the cellar.

I was expecting to meet someone whose sense of humour and sense of fun made her loveable but now I know a bit more I am quite proud to be part of the devotion she deserves in the final, chaotic years of her life. Respect? No problem.

One or two of Zuscha's more incomprehensible habits fall into place once you know some of this. Such as the hours spent watching people's comings and goings out of the window from behind a patch of curtain, wondering what everyone might be up to. And the basement door obsession, it must be checked behind, locked and bolted on a regular basis. One of my regular jobs is to check that we haven't imprisoned a stray workman or trapped one of the cats.

We have two cats by the way. They're both called Misha. We have a big Misha cat and a little Misha cat. Easy. And for reasons that are lost in the mists of time, as far as Zuscha is concerned, they are both good doggies. My day generally begins with the house echoing to the strains of the incomparably delightful line 'Hello Misha cat, are you a good doggie?' affectionately bellowed from one end of the hallway to the other. It's good to start the morning with a grin. Even if we have beaten dawn by several hours.

Pat has stayed with us for the first week or so, which means that I can filter into the routine rather than spend my days glued to pieces of paper full of notes. There are special diets and medications to get the hang of for a start and light-hearted tricks for getting both food and tablets consumed with minimum confrontation.

Ways too of getting a nicotine patch adhered somewhere it is unlikely to be found without mentioning cigarettes. Zuscha has always smoked. It's hard to be denied such an innocent pleasure when there's little else left to enjoy in life but forgetting you have a lit cigarette in your hand isn't safe for any of us. Any mention of cigarettes sets her off wanting to smoke one right away. This is OK from time to time, we have a few set aside for those days when diversion just isn't going to work but the attention required to spot the moment a cigarette is forgotten and dispose of it safely is pretty labour-intensive. There is no specific health reason to deny the nicotine though, in fact Pat has read research to show that it can actually be quite good for the cognitive connections that Alzheimer's destroys. The patches do seem to help with cognition as well as craving; on days when she finds the patch and removes it she has much more trouble interpreting the world, so the subterfuge is definitely worth a little time, effort and inventiveness.

There are favourite meals to learn and special recipes. Mainly involving psyllium husks. I understand that these fab little chaps are miraculous with regard to regularity. I'm learning the whereabouts of all the various drugstores and health food shops for buying said husks and a load of other terribly healthy and alternative things I've never heard of and didn't know anyone needed.

Most important of all, I'm learning Zuscha's favourite haunts for sitting and drinking coffee and watching the world go by. We peoplewatch a lot. Zuscha watches the children and the good doggies and I watch the men. Who all seem to be sporting mullets to go with their pot-bellies. And the obligatory baseball cap. Coming from a land where only adolescents and tourists favour this particular form of fashion statement – forwards or backwards – I find them fascinating. I am particularly charmed by the elderly couples with baseball hats that match. With or without mullets. There are tee-shirts to watch as well. Now correct me if I'm wrong but it seems to me that no self respecting Brit since the 60s has voluntarily sported a souvenir tee shirt of England. It's just about permissible to wear one from somewhere flash if you've been there on holiday but here, the maple leaf sits snugly over bellies of such amazing variety that my eyes are permanently riveted to people's wobbly bits.

What is my new job all about? Learning recipes, shopping lists and favourite cafes? Sitting about all day drinking coffee and viewing the general public as a cabaret just for us? Playing cat and mouse with chocolate in shops and admiring pebbles? Well yes mainly but that's the easy bit, the stuff that shows. There is a subtext; my real job is to try and generate an equal partnership, friendly and safe with some dignity attached. Anyone can tell Zuscha what to do all day and shovel medications down her; helping her to feel in charge of things, enabling her to make decisions and feel significant, that's the challenge. And on days when I'm not being disingenuously naïve about transatlantic culture I can be enough of an 'ologist to find the challenge fascinating and fun.

Opinion on the best way to handle Alzheimer's seems to polarise into two basic camps, there's Reality Orientation and there's Validation. Pat is my boss and Validation is what she wants. It involves changing some of the rules we tend to live by, rejigging the things that are supposed to matter and seeing the world a little differently. Through Alzheimer's eyes in fact. Starting with the assumption that – on the inside – there is some kind of logic to be made of everything Zuscha says or does, however bizarre it may appear. If you can't see what it means you're not thinking hard enough. No arguing or confrontation, if you can't work it out yet you look for the underlying emotion and work with that until the penny drops. In Zuscha's world she is running her family home, we are guests and her husband will be home later. Why the hell should she go to the toilet just because I tell her to? Reality is irrelevant. There are no calendars in our world and very few names. If it doesn't matter what day it is, it doesn't matter whether you know what day it is. It will only be distressing that you don't know who I am if I appear to care that you don't know who I am. If Zuscha smiles when she sees me, that's a bonus.

'I think I know you.'

'I think I know you too, maybe we met somewhere.'

'Maybe.'

'Shall we eat breakfast?'

An easy-going, confrontation-free day involves treating Zuscha much as many women treat their menfolk, i.e. letting her think it was her idea all along, although at times when a stand-off is inevitable it's easier to anticipate and defuse trouble before it happens than to trick your way out of it after it has. Which brings us neatly back to the dandelion.

Zuscha adores her 'yellow ones'. She spends hours collecting them from our lawn. And the neighbours' lawns. And the park, car parks, municipal flower beds, highway hard shoulders – nowhere is sacred. Once thoroughly established in a flowerbed of course, she pulls out everything else as well but dandelions are extra special.

Steffi (next door to the left and very nice about her denuded borders) had her lawn sprayed with pesticide yesterday. There was a little warning notice about keeping off, washing hands and other noxious chemical musts. And a big fat juicy dandelion right where you could see it from our kitchen window. Zuscha doesn't do musts or handwashings. Will we have the stand-off or the trip to hospital? Sneaking out at nap time to snaffle the culprit was a staggering piece of forethought for which my pride was all-consuming.

I celebrated by buying Ben a baseball hat with the Toronto Raptors on it. He likes the name because raptors are a type of dinosaur. We really must find out whether they play hockey, baseball or basketball but it's a rather embarrassingly stupid question to ask anybody. I'm on 'keeping a sharp eye on the sports pages' detail until we work it out for ourselves. Oh and it looks like we're staying.

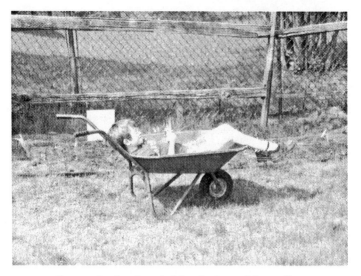

Ben settles in, denuded borders notwithstanding

FOUR

Flying solo

Pat has gone home and my laptop has died. I'm not sure which of these crises is the more traumatic. I was expecting to feel somewhat anxious during my first few days in sole charge on Planet Alzheimer but wasn't prepared for the agony of being prevented from writing a cheery missive about it to email home. The diary is becoming an obsession, my only escape. It began when Laura returned to the UK, I seem to need a running commentary now and have to write it down since she isn't here to film it. This isn't a good week to be incommunicado.

Shouting at Ben is a poor substitute but I'm doing it anyway. He takes it well. 'It's all right Mum, I know you're a bit stressed' but it seems rather mean, why should a kid have to understand about stress? He is already having to understand more about the smellier aspects of Alzheimer's than I had envisaged and we are both learning that when Ben and Zuscha both need attention at the same time, he's the only one of the pair who can comprehend that someone is just going to have to wait. He gets shouted at then too.

Fortunately since all his friends have now taken him home to charm their parents with his accent he's rarely without an invitation to go somewhere else and get away from his faintly frantic mother.

Zuscha and I rub along OK more often than not. She spent a couple of days putting her hat and coat on from time to time and heading for the bus stop, looking for Pat I think. This is easier to handle now I've learned the trick for turning her round without a fight when she's determined to leave home. You walk alongside her quietly for a few minutes until it starts to feel like a joint expedition. Then you sort of decide together that you're a bit cold, tired, thirsty, or whatever and maybe we could pop back for a coat/rest/drink and come back to the bus stop later. Once the decision to nip home for something is a mutual one, a biscuit as you walk back in through the door completes the manoeuvre and all is peace again. She has stopped going to get the bus now and is beginning to introduce me to people as her daughter.

The computer is doing less well. It is utterly deceased and I have finally had to bite the visa card and buy a new one, despite strenuous efforts on its behalf by a charming bunch of chaps in a tiny computer repair shop that I found in the phone book. Gosh these Canadians are friendly. They sat me in a corner and plied me with coffee, doughnuts, beer and amusing conversation while pursuing a mission to restore me to cyberspace. For a short while the problem seemed to resolve itself and I was able to email again. Surprisingly enough the first email I received was from one of the aforementioned computer repair chappies. Would I like to go out one day for more coffee and doughnuts and possibly beer and amusing conversation? I was terribly proud of myself. My first transatlantic proposition. I'd have been a lot prouder if it had come from the chap I had rather fancied as opposed to the older and less appealing sidekick but at my age it's definitely the principle that counts.

I opted for the ongoing feeble excuse gambit rather than an outright refusal. Well, the computer might require more attention so I couldn't afford to offend anyone could I? Besides, a girl needs a hobby. This turned out to be an extremely ill-judged decision. The feebler my excuses became, the grander this chap's plans for our non-existent relationship. Just at the point where he was going to whisk me off to Niagara Falls for a romantic weekend, I realised that I was going to have to start learning to use a very different form of communication. Canadians appear to be more American than British when it comes to hints.

Back home, an excuse whose feebleness is blatant enough serves as a polite 'no thanks'. Brits know where they are with feeble excuses, they read between the lines, they peruse the subtext. They guess that you are unlikely to be washing your hair or defleaing the cat every evening for a week. They appreciate your tact and diplomacy and move on. It would be terribly rude and unnecessarily forthright to say to a British potential beau 'I would prefer not to date you thanks very much.' Now just in case you are Canadian and male I shall insert a word of advice here – if you are dealing with a British woman, she is unlikely to want your assistance with cat defleament. She's being tactful.

Where was I? oh yes, since courteous evasion didn't appear to be working in my favour, I decided to give silence a try before doing the unthinkably un-British thing and telling him in words of one syllable that he wasn't going to take me anywhere. Then the computer died again. Silent evasion no longer an option. The unthinkable not only vital but urgent. After a complicated day of phone calls and a lot of trying not to give the wrong impression, I ended up minus my first Canadian admirer and plus a second-hand laptop procured for me most reasonably by another of the coffee and doughnut boffins. I think they're all still talking to me but it's hard to tell. What with everyone being so polite and all.

* * *

We've had a Bank Holiday. For Victoria Day. It's news to me but apparently the 24th of May is Queen Victoria's birthday. The nation celebrates with gusto and sets off fireworks in her honour. People are surprised to hear that we don't honour the good lady in this way at home. When I explain that we don't waste our fireworks on Royalty, we save them for the chap who tried but failed to blow up parliament, they think I am joking; that this is my equivalent of the pumpkin hunting myth. I know that Guy Fawkes Day is as real as Groundhog Day but it sounds equally unlikely when you start to try and explain.

While I am researching bank holidays and the inadvisability of not saying what I mean, Ben has been investigating the wildlife. He met a racoon this week. It was scuffling about in our neighbour's dustbin, sorry, garbage can. Apparently they can get nasty if they think you're between them and food (raccoons not neighbours) so he was advised to step away very carefully to avoid being bitten. Did you know that they have prehensile thumbs? Raccoons, not neighbours. Well, obviously the neighbours do as well but that's not the point. Our garbage can has a sort of wire clip to keep the lid on because of foraging fauna. The racoons just take it off anyway. Groundhogs can't do this, so the raccoons take the lids off, knock the bins over, eat what they fancy and leave the rest for the groundhogs.

And what's more, if you run over a skunk (which fortunately we haven't yet) you need to wash the car tyres in tomato juice to get rid of the smell. It's something to do with enzymes. Can't wait to try it out. But maybe not just yet awhile, there is always the possibility that someone is having me on. Is this one a Groundhog Day or a Pumpkin

Hunt? Trying to fathom which pieces of advice are genuine and which are the spoofs is becoming a major headache. For example, when we went to Toronto for the day (our first proper sight seeing trip; London, Ontario didn't count, we went, bought postcards, came home, it's not a hugely exciting destination) I decided to chicken out of driving there. It wasn't just the prospect of running over a skunk on the highway, people kept telling us how terrible, congested and confusing the traffic in the big city would be so we went by Greyhound bus instead.

Going somewhere by Greyhound should form part of the transatlantic experience I reasoned, besides it would be daft to risk our necks in scary traffic let alone spend hard earned cash on tomato juice. When we finally hit town (you are naturally way ahead of me here) it had nothing on a typical drive in London. Was it a deliberate con? Difficult to say, Canada is pretty empty, maybe Toronto streets do feel congested to a local. Either way I will drive next time, wildlife notwithstanding.

While we were there we did all the things real tourists should. A trip up the CN Tower, a walk on the glass floor (well, Ben did that bit while I hung onto the wall on the other side of the room) a trip round the harbour, too much ice cream. I suddenly felt extremely clever. There we sat, by Lake Ontario, writing postcards from somewhere I had never imagined we'd be able to afford to visit. We'd got there with a bit of wit, a lot of hard work and a smidgeon of being brave. I came over all soppy and hugged the pair of us for being so brilliant.

Then it was time for a quick play on the streetcars and home to see how Zuscha had coped without me. Or rather, how the nice lady from the Red Cross who replaced me for the day had coped with Zuscha. They appeared to have had a relatively peaceful time, which bodes well for more days off. Zuscha seems to save up major naughtiness for me. Is this a good thing? I think possibly it is.

* * *

There was a very apologetic knock at the door later that evening. Apparently our next-door neighbour is planning to sell his house. Some potential buyers were on their way to view the place and Zuscha was happily installed in their flower beds on a root-snaffling mission. I've no idea how she got there, she must have sneaked out while I had a wee. She's like greased lightning when you're not looking and there's a dandelion to be had. Anyway, his thesis was that a batty old lady resident in the foliage might have a detrimental effect on the asking price and could I help at all? I lured her away with a particularly scrumptious biscuit and then lurked in the foliage myself trying to render the gates inoperative with a stray bit of wire, while keeping out of sight of both Zuscha and potential buyers. I'm becoming the local garden fugitive.

Ben is having a bit of a hard time coping with Zuscha's more difficult ways. He can't quite understand why an adult should get away with behaving so badly when he can't. He also fumes quietly when she tries to 'look after him', which of course she does because he is a kid and she is a Mum. Nights irritate him the most. She wanders a lot and understandably gets a bit confused as to who is sleeping where, so she does a regular check on all the bedrooms. I had an old German Shepherd dog once that did the same. Only he couldn't turn the light on.

We've taken the light bulb out of Ben's room now and put a big notice on the door that says 'Shh, Ben is sleeping in here.' So now she stops outside his door, reads the note at a low bellow, looks in and yells 'are you asleep?' He is almost amused by the fact that if he says 'yes' she goes away quite happy.

Less antisocial antics delight him though and he does like to be first to investigate the cats' bowls in the morning. Another of Zuscha's nightly rituals is the feeding of the cats. It's anybody's guess what will be in the bowl in the morning and he is compiling a list. Often there will be the remains of the tempting but wholesome midnight feast I 'accidentally' leave lying about to fuel her nightly wanderings. Some soggy bran biscuits perhaps or meticulously shaved pear peelings. Most spectacular were the jigsaw puzzle pieces spread carefully with jam, although the bowl of *Coolwhip* amused us greatly too. This stuff is a little like *Dream Topping*. It has been the subject of much controversy among the stable of respite carers who fill in here from time to time. So much had been disappearing from the fridge that each had accused the others of taking it home. I think I can now identify the culprit. Maybe I should tell them.

Our whole days off are pretty rare but thanks to these long-suffering ladies we do get two or three hours out of the house once or twice a week. Long enough enjoy the fact that there is a park full of trees just round the corner and to work on our favourite doughnut. We are used of course to doughnuts which come with jam in. Or without jam in. The idea of several chains of shops dedicated to the humble doughnut struck us as a little absurd – until we walked into one. You name it, it comes in a doughnut. They are a continual source of delight and surprise. It's just as well we have two years, it'll take that long to choose a favourite.

Just when I thought I was on top of things, Zuscha had a bad week. There are no adjectives adequate for the quality of my week. She was much more disorientated than usual, ergo, even more weeding. It was impossible to divert her from her chosen flowerbed to eat or drink, put on a coat or get out of the sun. She was as overtired as a toddler and sleeping in restless fits and starts. With even more broken nights than usual I was exhausted too. She managed to launch an escape

51

attempt from her lunchtime day centre, which was a huge blow as she had seemed to be quite enjoying it there. We were just beginning to discuss increasing her hours from an experimental hour-on-a-Tuesday (which would have made for handy sleeping time for me) but it was not to be. I tried pointing out that she had merely spied a juicy dandelion out of the window and offered to pick them all myself as soon as we arrived next time so it wouldn't happen again but they don't have the staff to cope with absconders. So that little wheeze is on hold for a while and I've lost my much-needed little break.

On the day I wondered if I could take any more – shaking from lack of sleep I'd lost a contact lens – I made a momentous discovery. She likes watching cartoons on the TV. Ben was watching some Saturday morning children's junk, it caught her eye and she sat in one place for a whole two hours. So did I. It was bliss. I was a little worried that Pat wouldn't approve. It's not exactly active stimulation for the brain but she had a happy smile on her face and at 76 it must be vaguely beneficial to sit down for a while instead of walking about bent double all day hunting dandelions. I've started putting cartoons on when she wakes from her morning nap in an effort to keep her out of the sun when it's hottest.

I finally confessed to Pat during one of our weekly telephone bulletins and awaited disapproval. 'Well,' she said 'if she's happy and resting and not out getting dehydrated, what more can an old lady ask?' I am off the hook and we're all sleeping better again.

With a bit more sleep under my belt I perked up enough to attempt an evening out. I spent it at Kitchener's one and only comedy club. More weirdness, I'm trying to work out why. Firstly there are the plush surroundings, I'm used to grotty back rooms in nasty pubs. Then there are the twin odd concepts of people expecting a formal evening out and anticipating being amused during it. Not only was there a full dinner menu and waitress service but these folks were there to laugh. The comics didn't have to fight for every giggle from an audience determined to make them suffer. Instead of half a dozen hopefuls, desperate to succeed and more likely to die on their feet than win over the crowd, we had two professional comedians who clearly didn't mind whether the evening was a blast or not. Everyone laughed politely in all the right places. Was it the silent, stubborn defiance that I missed? The absence of passive aggression? Is it normal to assume that if it says Comedy Club outside you are probably going to laugh? Possibly.

I learned one or two of the cruder phrases they use here mind, and not before time. It's easy to be unwittingly ruder than you intend. (Ben learned very early on to use an eraser at school and I have been told never to knock him up in the morning.) Luckily I have the chaps at the computer shop to put me straight on such matters.

Yes, I've been back. The superduper little new computer required some tweaking. So, back I went for advice and repairs, and have had some very pleasant little chats over a beer or two with the scrumptious chap who initially caught my eye. I might have to drop in with a few return beers sometime. Just to express my gratitude for all the technical help you understand. Oh, the Raptors play basketball.

FIVE

Only in books

We are beginning to plan our first trip home. It's almost June, the wedding approaches and we have a fortnight's holiday to fly home, finish the cake, go to the wedding and generally show off. It's hard to believe we've been here two months and Pat is preparing to pop back and cover for our first allotted break. We are both happily looking forward to seeing friends and family again because in the main, we are more pleased with ourselves than homesick. I do wonder though how flying back to Toronto a second time will feel. It won't be a venture into the unknown this time, we are as aware of the tough bits as we are as of the excitement.

I think Ben will be OK, he is heading for a summer of camps and pals and all-day bike rides (come home when it gets dark or if you get hungry, whichever happens first, how very Enid Blyton) but I know now that my summer will consist of running round in the sun chasing Zuscha out of people's gardens, tipping bucket loads of weeds off the kitchen table to make room for every meal and laundering a lot of wet underwear.

Carolyn Steele

I cope most of the time and the good times definitely outweigh the bad; as I write this I am sitting in the *el-nino* sponsored unseasonable sunshine – you should see my tan, I've never had one before – watching a Blue Jay hop about on the lawn. It occurs to me that there are worse ways to work your way across a country, wet knickers notwithstanding. And anyway, the next big adventure is looming, driving the Trans Canada Highway to transfer Zuscha to British Columbia. Unmissable, of course I will be eager to return.

Please be impressed that I knew it was a Blue Jay by the way. Bird watching is not a passion of mine but it's hard not to take a slight interest here, they're all so big. The aforementioned Blue Jays are violently blue. They make up for the spectacular plumage by letting themselves down a little in the singing department. This particular chap squawks outside my bedroom window shortly before good-doggie time every morning, a sound reminiscent of a strangled crow with temporary charge of a foghorn. There are times when prettiness is just no excuse. Robins are at least twice the size of any I've seen before, with redder, perkier breasts than ever graced a Christmas card and every so often a huge scarlet effort appears in the garden as well. A Cardinal I think. I'm almost looking forward to seeing my first Chickadee. Back to Hollywood, I never knew chickadees were birds before. I thought they were just, well, you know, terms of endearment.

It is possible that I'm burbling about birds in order to put off the next topic of conversation, I've almost been on a date you see. There's unexpected for you. My opportunity to return all those beers cropped up when my new computer hero suggested we joined him and his son at the local 'Laser Quest' emporium. The idea being that the kids could run about and shoot each other and he and I could sit in the bar and drink beer. I'm not sure if it counts as a date if the children go too but it will do my ego good to call it such;

56

and since we had a good time and may do it again I shall preen a few feathers and forget about the semantics.

Of course, the last thing I need just now is to get all wound up about whether some bloke is going to pick the phone up or not. Not in the intrepid game plan at all, I can do that at home. So despite the fact that I've 'met someone' as my mother would put it, I'm resolutely not going to care whether I see him again or not. I've notched up another invitation for the record and that's the end of it. Anyway, travelling all this way just to end up doing something sissy like falling in love only happens to people in books.

Computer Hero may be a complication and possible source of soppy diary entries but in my defence, he is also good source of suggestions for places to visit and, thus advised and inspired Ben and I went for another little drive about at the weekend. We like our little drives about, you never know what you're going to find next. Apart from a doughnut shop even better than the last. On this occasion we headed off in search of a cheese shop which we never found. What we found instead was another unpredictable Canadian institution, vending machines for live fishing bait. Somehow *Best Worms. Fresh Spawn* seemed a little distasteful on the harmless machine I leant against while finishing an ice cream. How do they stay alive in a sealed metal box? Well I assume it's sealed otherwise there would have been worms all over the road. Do they need oxygen? I don't know. And what is a substandard worm? Do I want to think about this any more? Not really. I'll just be a bit more careful where I lean in future.

And so will Ben, we hadn't been back half an hour when he had a nasty fall. His patent device to defeat Zuscha's chocolate divining antennae involves placing his tuck box on a high shelf inside a cupboard in his room. He was climbing on a chair to reach for it when he and the chair took a tumble. Zuscha and I both heard the crash. We both made for his room and when she saw him in a heap on the floor crying, Zuscha realised what had happened. For a moment she was most concerned. Then she spied a piece of fluff on the floor and the moment passed.

Ben had landed heavily on one arm and was in obvious pain, Zuscha, bent double and obliviously intent on fluff, occupied the space between him and me. 'Please get her out of here Mum.' I tried. But the fluff on the floor was very important. I shouldn't have shouted but I did. Zuscha left Ben's room, put her coat on, picked up several handbags and headed off to the bus stop.

Well what would you do first? I really needed to give Ben's arm a thorough examination and possibly take him to hospital. I also really needed to comfort a rejected old lady who was leaving home because I'd shouted at her. Suddenly it wasn't a game I was OK at playing most of the time, it was an impossible mix of terrifying responsibilities totally incompatible with one other. This wouldn't be the only time the mix would explode, if I sorted this one out there'd be another and there wouldn't be time to sit down and cry then either.

In the time it took Zuscha to find her shoes (thank goodness she remembered them) I gave the injured arm the full ambulanceman's once-over (can you move it luv?) before turning my attention to the injured ego. The arm looked OK, had it been anyone else's son my advice would have been to stick a bag of frozen peas on it and worry if it turned purple in the morning. But this was Ben. A part of me really wanted to get it x-rayed anyway.

While wielding the emergency peas, I persuaded Zuscha to have a cup of coffee before she went to catch the bus. And actually, I could take her where she wanted to go in the car in the morning, which might be nicer because it was getting dark and cold. We all calmed down eventually. And it didn't turn purple in the morning. Makes you think though. I have

a list of phone numbers of friendly neighbours now, ready
for the next emergency. I have also resolved to be less cocky
next time I'm asked how I'm coping.

* * *

We've seen Niagara Falls. No really. Isn't that amazing?
I don't quite know which I found more breathtaking, the
sight of those never-ending walls of water, or the fact that
we'd come all this way and managed to see them. That
sensation is getting to be a habit. We stayed for the weekend
which means that we were there overnight. Yes, I know
that's obvious but the point is, when we went back to gawp
at the Falls again on the morning of our second day, *they
were still going*. I couldn't get over this. Where does it all
come from? The geographical answer just doesn't work. I
was going to say doesn't wash but this is no time for puns.
I must have used the word awesome sometime in my life
before but now I actually know what it means.

The town itself is extremely touristy and full of tacky
ways to part you from your money. Canadians are quite
sniffy about it being so down-market, a little like Londoners
on the subject of all those vulgar souvenir vendors who
spoil so many of our more august national monuments
by having the temerity to earn a living. But nothing could
possibly spoil this view. Not for me anyway, I could sit
there and dream for days. And anyway, as I said to those
who predicted disappointment ('it's only water') we don't
have big geography at home.

We do however have the teletubbies, don't we? There's
a big hoo-ha here over the teletubbies. Not their educational
value or lack of it but their language. Cuddly tubby toys
have hit the shelves and they say things when you press
their tummies. Apparently to Transatlantic ears it sounds as
though Po is saying *faggot* when you press his tum. Strongly

worded letters have been written to the papers about two year olds learning such seditious stuff.

According to the manufacturers Po is actually saying *fidit* which is Cantonese for faster. The original Po was a Cantonese actress who introduced the term while having a fun time on Po's scooter. More strongly worded letters to the papers about how a two-year-old could mistake one word for the other unless already attuned to such filth by its parents. This delicious row looks set to run until Christmas. I am keeping cuttings.

Have I strayed off topic? Are my musings a little random? Welcome to Planet Alzheimer Carolyn, leave your train of thought at immigration and make yourself at home. Where was I? Oh yes…

We had our weekend off courtesy of Pat who is back to cover for our trip home. I was a little apprehensive that she would arrive during a down part of Zuscha's ups and downs and hold me responsible but she seems quite happy with what she has found here and I am mightily relieved. I can fly home a little more confident that I'm an adequate sidekick, give or take the odd elbow, which may make it easier to come back. It'll be a summer full of dandelion hunts all right but we do now definitely have the Big Move to look forward to.

Pat's plans are progressing well. She is building us a new house. Pat is apparently an old hand at such things and she is building, on Saltspring Island, an exact replica of the house we live in now, with all the rooms in the same places so that Zuscha will always be able to find the bathroom. Then we will all move together to live next door to Pat, ready for when I have served my time. It will take a year of residency in British Columbia before Zuscha can qualify for any provincial assistance but after that time Pat thinks she will be able to manage with local respite carers.

Quite how Zuscha will react to her habitual home suddenly having a new view is anybody's guess of course and – much though I don't want to look a gift job in the mouth – it does all seem a bit Heath-Robinson as a way to take care of one's parent. When Pat first came to England I rather assumed she was Zuscha's only child but apparently there is another, a brother. He and his wife live about a mile from here. According to Pat neither of them of them is quite up to the task of caring for Zuscha properly. They send her birthday cards, which is thoughtless and not very Validation. Be that as it may (and I resolutely refuse to even consider developing an opinion of my own over such a politically sensitive issue) it sheds a slightly different light on the NATO style planning that has gone into the importing of me and the building of replica house.

I find the consideration and energy that have gone in to the whole enterprise rather humbling and I hope someone loves me that much when I'm old and difficult; but I do wonder whether I've stumbled into a life-sized sibling rivalry game. And if I have, for how long will keeping my mouth shut and doing as I am told keep me out of the firing line? Will there be tears before bed-time? I am beginning to understand why Pat had to look abroad for her stand-in.

SIX

Another sad fool running away?

We're in London – London, England. On holiday. We're not happy. How come we never knew how nasty it was before? Dirty streets and buildings, litter, graffiti, traffic and noise. The noise is the worst part. Home can't have been deafening before can it? Surely we'd have noticed. Although, come to think of it, I remember Rachael returning from Australia and saying 'it's so noisy I can't hear you' and I didn't understand. Now I'm walking out of shops without the things I need, in order to escape the wall of sound.

The noise may be bad but the faces are worse. Everyone looks tense, stressed, angry. I want to go home. We're missing our new friends, we both feel closer to them than old ones. It's a bizarre sensation, recognising where you are but feeling like a stranger anyway. Ben finally said it for both of us, 'Why don't I feel as though I've lived here all my life?' Me? I'm still trying to turn the volume down.

Meeting old pals is surreal. The first comment everyone makes is 'My God you look well!' And we do but I get the feeling one or two would prefer it if we didn't. Then there are all the questions. I thought I wanted to tell all but it's hard to know where to start. And then when we do, we're not telling it how people want to hear it. We seem to be expected to cheer people up by telling them the stories they have in their heads. I'm racing about at everyone's beck and call, saying the same meaningless things time and again and resenting every moment.

I am only comfortable with people who have done it themselves. Cast adrift for a while, been 'away'. They are able to let me sit and say 'this is odd' as many times as I like. Rachael – who knows how noisy it is – and Mary, who belongs in New Zealand and endures being the cabaret during her own visits home. They have spared me 'what's the weather like then?' and 'I suppose the telly's crap eh?'

Mary put her finger on the other irritation for me. Everybody else is still living the same life they were ploughing through when we left. You expect for some irrational reason that because your world has changed, everyone else will have moved on too; whereas in reality the school PTA politics are the same, this one's boyfriend troubles and that one's medical symptoms are – word for word – as they were when we left. Almost as though it's all been stored in mental mothballs for me to unpack as soon as I'm back in my old pigeonhole. I must be stressed, I'm mixing metaphors again. I'll be burning juggernauts any minute.

All things considered, the wedding cake is coming along remarkably well. Despite the jet-lag. Funny stuff jet-lag. We both started off tired, slept it off and thought it was over. Then the ambush sets in, suddenly getting the shakes in the middle of the day because your body thinks it's five in the morning and you have worked enough of your night shift. Getting up seven times a night to wee because your bladder thinks it's day time. I'm told you should allow a day for each hour of time difference before attempting anything complicated. So I probably started on the old sugar orchids and iced *broderie anglais* a little early. It'll be done for the big day of course. Nicky has seen it almost finished and it was good to see her smile. I finally felt as though I might manage to enjoy the wedding, so I decided to risk a trip up the ladder to retrieve my only decent jacket from the loft. (The lodgers kindly made temporary room for us back in the old house.) Made it safely up and down. Found jacket. Slipped refolding ladder and hit self in mouth with same. I now have a fat lip for the photos. Have made diligent efforts with the emergency frozen peas but still look as though I have taken up boxing. Have realised that it's not so much me not liking ladders as them not liking me.

Meanwhile, Ben has been mobbed. He sneaked up to his old school and lurked outside his class at turning out time. The resultant jubilation took him completely by surprise. He has subsequently put his finger on an idea that I hadn't quite developed yet. We've been missing our friends a bit but have been too busy doing new things to miss them as much as they have missed us. His perceptiveness staggers me at times. And I feel even meaner for resenting something in my own friends that Ben can view with magnanimity at the age of nine. Travel may not be broadening my mind much but at this rate he'll be a philosopher by next year.

* * *

The wedding was lovely but then that's what they are for. Suited and booted and hatted and blending into the fuzzy photos of friends-of-the-bride, in the Englishest of surroundings, we ate and drank and laughed just as though we were normal. No-one cared who we were or where we'd been because Nicky was on stage today. Almost as much of a relief as a cake which tasted as good as it looked. It had been most competently brandied and the sugar orchids behaved

65

impeccably, staying in one piece despite road works on the A1(M) so I didn't once need to resort the superglue secreted in my handbag. Do all cake makers attend weddings with superglue in their handbags? Probably. I was even offered a job. The dress designer – sorry, wedding stylist – who normally 'themes society functions my dear' declared that she would 'love me on board'. I'd forgotten how pretentious we Brits could be. It felt good to be able to say, 'Much though I'd love to be on board as your cake stylist, sadly I'm leaving the country next week.' Have sneaked her phone number away though, just in case I'm in need of income when we return. Might have to edit 'pretentious' out. Just in case.

And I think I know what's been wrong. Another big relief. Two months is long enough to feel at home in Canada, to have friends and social lives and want to go back. We're missing people and sending postcards, which makes us feel all clever and settled but it's not long enough for me to have outgrown all the things I tried to leave behind. Particularly my house. I don't want it to be my home any more, it's full of a failed marriage and wasted dreams. The moment I walked through the door it was like putting on an old coat and suddenly remembering the time you got caught in the rain in it. Now I'm wondering if we've moved ourselves all that way just for me to try and leave my bitter memories too far behind to retrieve. If so, it clearly hasn't worked. Maybe I'm not a bold adventurer after all, just another sad fool running away from myself and then finding that I took myself along for the ride. Heady stuff for a holiday ponder but possibly better out than in. On the bright side, at least there's no danger of not wanting to go back to work. I'm missing Zuscha.

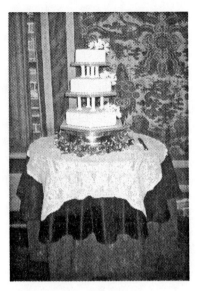

The orchids behaved impeccably

Thank goodness for trivia. I've found a lighter ponder to keep the soul-searching at bay. I've been musing on the question of time travel. It began when I decided to keep Canadian time on my laptop so that I could see when to expect return emails. As I sit emailing across the Pond late at night – well, early in the morning really – and send a message back five hours, in effect from today to yesterday, I can't quite work out where the intervening hours have gone. Why doesn't changing your watch on the plane produce the same amazement? Or asking people what the time is 'over there' on the phone? It's the same trick after all. Maybe because one does it less frequently, with other things to think about at the time. Sending messages from screen to screen is still a tad novel to a technophobe like me I suppose, so the idea that I'm writing to the past and that other people are writing to the future is utterly mind blowing. Where are those hours? The only reason I didn't lose five hours of my life for ever when we flew here is because I'll get them back again when we return. Maybe I just have a 'little country' mentality. Canada spans so many time zones, everyone else probably got used to it in their cradle.

Here's a confession. When I say 'emailing my chums' I really mean emailing Computer Hero. To my eternal shame, I'm missing him a bit too much for comfort. With emails time-travelling equally often in both directions it's possible I'm not the only one. Plans are afoot for a celebratory drink on my return. Maybe I am writing a book after all.

We went to Covent Garden on our last day, looking for nicely tacky souvenirs of London to take back for our new Canadian pals. We found a talking Po in *Hamleys*. We both listened carefully and I have to say that he (she?) definitely does say faggot. The little minx. I think I'll write to the papers.

* * *

Flying into Toronto this time was no less exciting, just a bit different. Ben spotted the CN Tower from the plane. The idea that somewhere in Canada could be familiar from the air bowled us both over. Maybe we really were coming home. And just in time for Canada Day. More fireworks. Darned decent gesture we thought, to celebrate our return in such style. We decided to attend the nearest birthdayfest in an effort to stay awake until normal going-to-bed time. My yardstick for firework displays has long been Alexandra Palace on Guy Fawkes Day. These matched up pretty well and Ben bawled out *Oh Canada* with the best of them. After a term of singing it each morning at school (now isn't that strange?) he can do both verses with gusto. The only damper on the proceedings was the time it took to get home.

I've not encountered a traffic jam here before. Judging by the time it took the local police to sort out some marshals neither has anyone else. Fifty-five thousand people attended this particular Canada Day extravaganza. The sensible ones walked there. The rest of us sat for one-and-a-half hours waiting to get out of the car park. And I mean waiting. No-one swore or shouted, no-one hooted a horn, no-one got out of their car to have words with the guy at the front who actually couldn't go anywhere anyway. We waited. Had this been Harringay, blood would have spilled in the first ten minutes. Flabbergasted, I mentioned this to Pat the following day. She told us the standard Canadian joke:

'How do you get twenty-five Canadians out of a swimming pool?'

'You ask them nicely to get out now please.'

Since we're calling K/W home, it behoves me to describe our home town. I should call it a city, or more properly a twin-city, but I have trouble using either epithet for anywhere that can get its street map onto one sheet of paper and doesn't have a cathedral.

Kitchener and Waterloo are two cities sharing a border, effectively the same place. Each has its own 'downtown' area, city centre to you and me. They are a few miles apart on the same through road. Waterloo, being to the north, likes to call its downtown uptown. Suburban streets fill the gaps between the down-uptowns and the various shopping malls dotted around the edges. People look after their lawns a lot. Waterloo has universities and considers itself the intellectual wing of the outfit, so naturally sports a slightly trendier feel, vegetarian eateries and funky fair trade craft shops. Kitchener has the government offices – tax and immigration and the like – so considers itself the commercial engine room.

Waterloo sees Kitchener as no better than it ought to be, Kitchener sees Waterloo as every-so-slightly ivorytowerish. Kitchener has the nightclubs, Waterloo has the bookshop cafes. Either side of the border, everywhere is terrifyingly quiet. Shops and restaurants are permanently empty. There's nothing wrong with them, they're all very nice, there just aren't enough people to go round. The local paper is full of editorials on the subject of downtown (and uptown) regeneration; most blame the planners and call for more in-town cinemas and fewer out-of-town shopping malls.

Can you designate a town centre? Tell people where to congregate? There's just so much space that the available people won't fill anywhere unless they really want to. The answer seems to me to be to move the entire conurbation three paces to the right so that the Grand River runs through the centre of town rather than around the edge, people like to hang out along river banks. But I'm not a town planner so what do I know?

I'm getting used to eating in empty restaurants but can't handle empty bars yet. I miss pubs a bit. Getting happily tipsy is something best done in a crowded, preferably dingy environment. Big, bright, clean empty bars with extensive menus and waitress service just exude sobriety. I popped hopefully into a self-styled English Pub, to find a bright, clean, empty bar with waitress service and draft Guinness. It was called the *Fox and Pheasant* though, so that helped.

By way of a last project before Pat leaves me to it again, we have been fitting movement detectors around the house. The plan is that a bell will ring if Zuscha wanders too far afield. This might make it possible for me to use the bathroom sometimes without being scared of losing her. Since she travels fast and below window level on her weeding binges the detectors have to be set to pick up bent-over people as well as upright ones. Pat and I spent a happy afternoon crawling round the house on our hands and knees and ringing bells. Zuscha thinks we're nuts.

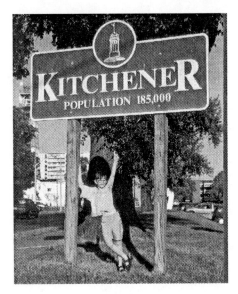

Where?

SEVEN

It rhymed with potato

Pat is back in British Columbia and we are back to normal. Zuscha seems to be a lot calmer than when we left, sleeping more, eating better and having conversations – occasionally with people. This perkiness could be due to an experimental drug regime she is taking part in. Every six months or so the wonder-stuff has to be administered by intravenous infusion, a dose each day for a fortnight. I've been learning about it as I'll be in charge of organising the next round of visiting nurses. The drug – when it works and it doesn't for everyone – takes several weeks to kick in and then lasts for four or five months, after which time her cognitive function deteriorates very fast. The most recent dose of this stuff (it doesn't have a name yet, being just a prototype) was happening when we first arrived here, so we are probably seeing the best effects of it now.

I am told that the first set of infusions, last year sometime, produced a really dramatic improvement. The next made a noticeable difference but wasn't quite as effective. We are in the results of the third round now and the pattern seems to be that each dose helps a little less than the one before. So this is as good as it gets. Lulled into a false sense of security, I left her to her own devices in the bathroom for a while. Came back to find her scrubbing mud from her hands with a razor. Ho hum.

On a slightly more normal note, I only got into the wrong side of the car once this week. Driving on different sides of the road became instinctive surprisingly fast, I was expecting excruciating moments of indecision in the middles of junctions but there are multiple cues to help you get it right, from the colour of the line down the middle of the road, through the arrangements of traffic lights, to the tiny unreadable size of the arrows designating a one-way street. It's a bit like learning two languages I think – not that I've tried, Brits don't do they?

There are excruciating moments of indecision but they happen in car parks. No cues, lines, signage or street furniture to tell you which language to adopt, so for the first few days I am a little risky to be around at either end of a journey. That is once I am in the car, the really hard thing is finding that steering wheel. I have taken to loitering for a minute or two and taking a gentle stroll around the car before getting in. I try to look as though I might just kick a tyre shortly so that no-one will know I'm trying to remember which side I'll find the woofers and tweeters.

It dawns on me that I haven't yet waxed lyrical about the joys of Canadian driving. The roads are so clear and the speed limit so low that driving is a totally effortless and stress-free experience. To a Londoner a drive through K/W is as refreshingly restful as forty winks in the afternoon. Some things took a little getting used to, like being allowed to turn right against a red light, a total absence of lane discipline, signage that never works the same way twice and toasting the other arm out of the window. Weirdest of all, the four-way stop. Right of way defaults to the person whose wheels pull to a complete stop before anyone else's do. It works, people eye each others wheels most attentively and the first to stop is courteously allowed to be the first to go. Should it be a photo finish, right of way defaults to the right. Easy enough to learn in theory but it never occurred to this London driver that anyone would stick to the rules sufficiently well for it to work. I can negotiate them a little better now I am not paralysed by amazement every time; and am a little quicker off the mark at traffic lights as well now I have twigged there will not be an amber light before I can go. Sometimes I even remember to turn right when they're red.

Now that it's approaching second nature, nothing can match the sheer glee of cruising about on almost empty roads with my little map, feeling as though I own the place. Once I've found the engine room and got in, obviously.

Canadian though I occasionally feel behind the wheel, there is one thing I still can't handle with equanimity and that is the whole vexed question of baseball caps. Yes, I know I've mentioned them, well whinged about them, before but I still don't get it, although I feel that I should by now. I can see the point of a hat in which to play baseball, it's sunny here and a chap needs a hat if he's to be out all afternoon being sporty. Even cricketers sport a head covering of some sort (the umpires often wear several) but when the cricket's over they take them off. Why are bars and shopping malls full of people who don't play baseball wearing the blessed things indoors, at night and back to front?

I sat in a bar – I've found one that sometimes has people in – and tried to work out the code. I think forwards means 'I could be a bit sporty actually, if I lost a few pounds' and backwards means 'I'd like you to think I'm a bit of a rebel.' Can't fathom sideways baseball cap, braces and tie though. It says 'I'm a bit of a pillock' to me but that's unlikely to be the intention.

I can however recommend sitting in a bar with a pen and paper watching people. Why the pen and paper? Well I've been researching what you need to do to be a real travel writer recently and it would appear that the correct thing is sit in a bar until all sorts of culturally curious nuggets of gold happen around you, then you write them down. It's not a bad way to spend an evening off, eventually curiosity gets the better of someone and they have to ask, then you get bought a beer. I met two amazing women that way the other night whom I initially took for mother and daughter. It turned out that the older lady was the girlfriend of the ex-husband of the younger, have you got that? It took me a while and I'll be asking questions later.

After a merry evening they rang for him to come and drive them both home. Insisting that he bought me a drink first naturally. In fact they'd have made him drive me home too but I took pity on him and declined. The poor man was just about to go to bed when they called, he'd changed back out of his pyjamas to turn out for them. I was most impressed.

Perhaps I'm not going to become Bill Bryson that way but the only other thing that I do with any regularity is sit in restaurants with Zuscha. No-one buys us beer but I suppose anecdotes of excruciating embarrassment and horticultural vandalism have their place. It used to be just artificial flower arrangements and poppy seed muffins that caused the trouble. (We rip the flowers off the arrangements and remove our dentures to get at every last little pesky seed. I still can't bring myself to return to the café where I accidentally precipitated the awful poppy seed faux-pas.) But the latest source of social agony? Zuscha has taken a major dislike to fat people. She has started pointing them out everywhere. It started in the Texas Barbecue and Grill, where we'd gone for her all-time favourite lunch, Western Omelette and Home Fries. Western omelettes have ham in but I don't know what

Home Fries are meant to be yet, I thought from the menu that they meant chips cut from potatoes rather than exuded from a machine but apparently these are Fresh Cut Fries. Home Fries look a bit like sauté potatoes. I must pluck up the courage to ask someone sometime.

Anyway, across the restaurant from us was an ample lady consuming a relatively ample meal. 'Look at her!' bawled Zuscha, 'She's eating like a horse, no wonder she's so fat.' This was but the beginning. We then followed a well-built lady across the road on our way back to the car after lunch. 'You've got a fat bottom lady' rang out and reverberated around the municipal maple trees. Determined not to be embarrassed this time and immensely proud of my quick thinking I saved the day with a jocular riposte:

'Yes I know, I think I need to eat fewer cookies.'

'Not you, her!'

I made a mental note to check out our future destinations for fat people as well as vulnerable flower arrangements in future and to sit Zuscha facing away from both if possible and went back to nursing the tail end of my first Canadian hangover. They aren't any different from the usual variety, poorly head and collywobbles seem pretty universal but the stuff you buy over the counter here to cure them with is terrifying.

I'll start at the beginning. Please don't think I've been teetotal since our arrival here, the occasional beer has indeed passed my lips. And I've discovered a pretty tolerable Sangiovese that comes in one-and-a-half litre bottles, perfect for those troubling evenings at home. In fact, three glasses of said plonk and Zuscha and I function at pretty much the same pace. We both go to bed giggling, which is good for domestic harmony. I should have the stuff included in my wages.

Anyway, the day before the day in question dawned hot, humid, sticky and disgusting. The air quality here has been pretty poor recently. Apparently the Lakes collect pollution from the States and various things to do with high pressure make sure that K/W suffers the worst of it, although I have to say it is nothing like the average day in London. I digress, it was too hot to eat much.

Having arranged to meet Computer Hero for a beer – almost a date again but we aren't quite calling it that yet – I ambled out in high spirits. Two hours and too many beers later I was composing an article in my somewhat befuddled mind along the lines of 'never been stood up before…didn't need to come all this way to find out what that's like…could have done that at home…mutter mutter grumble whinge…' when he appeared, full of apologies. Various things had conspired to delay him, none of which I could legitimately object to (especially since it wasn't quite a date) so several more beers joined the empty stomach. I think I'm in love by the way. Which is just as well because this is almost a book.

I digress again, I had brought with me from home some supplies of my beloved *Panadol Extra* but these had been exhausted by an early dose of flu and replaced by some stuff that a pharmacist told me was similar. I had to be told because even generic drug names are different this side of the Pond, which seems daft to me. In addition to that, everything is 'extra strength' because it is a cocktail of lots of other things which are written in very small print and have the wrong names. Over-the-counter cocktails presumably make for very efficient symptom relief in a land where no-one can get a family doctor, unless like me, you are allergic to almost every medication known to man even if you know what it's called.

I am the only person I know who's allergic to Prozac for goodness sake, so heaven knows what the magic extra ingredient in my new headache cure was but I spent a day and a half alternately vomiting and falling over all dizzy before the dratted stuff wore off. And it wasn't really much of a hangover. Forgive me for rambling on about headache pills, I know it's hardly in the league of sultry-sunsets-over-dappled-waters sort of travel writing or the culturally curious bar gossip sort but having trouble curing a headache was among the last things on my mind when I considered the possible hazards of transatlantic adventuring. So much less romantic than being eaten by bears.

It wasn't a good week for feeling below par either. One of my respite carers had a crisis in the family and had to go home for several days. I didn't realise quite how much I needed my little breaks until they weren't there. I get a little stir-crazy after two days without a breather and I'm now well into my fourth. If I have to admire one more bloody bird in one more sodding tree I'll explode. There's something infinitely challenging about spending twenty-four hours a day looking out for the welfare of someone who fights you every step of the way. As long as I get an hour or two off every couple of days it stays an interesting challenge but without a break each little battle starts to hurt. I end up resenting being treated like a monster because I'd like Zuscha to have a drink or some food or some shade, because otherwise she'll be ill. It's just not funny any more, especially when you can't remember the last uninterrupted night's sleep.

If it weren't for *Chapters* I'd be tearing my hair out. *Chapters* is almost as good as a rest. *Chapters* is a bookshop. Not any old bookshop you understand, this one is a little piece of heaven sent to bless the folks between *Harvey's Drive-in Breakfast* and *Canadian Tire Mufflers*. Imagine a bookshop where the decor invites you in, the signage helps you round and just when you've found an interesting book to peruse, a comfy sofa materialises. There aren't any signs on the sofas saying 'please sit down and read our books for free' but there may as well be. The staff put them away when you've finished.

Add the aroma of coffee, perfect air conditioning and hundreds of magazines in case you don't feel quite up to a book, oh and more sofas, and you have the recipe for a place I could happily live for ever. As could most of the rest of K/W. This place is so popular it sometimes gets almost crowded. I think of bookshops as places where you linger at your peril. Spend too long investigating a potential purchase and the staff will be ringing Social Services in case you've mistaken the establishment for a library and therefore need to keep warm. This place – they're a chain and they deserve to take over the world – doesn't just want your custom, it wants your soul and it has mine.

When Zuscha and I spend an afternoon there I can plant her in an armchair so soft and squidgy that she can't clamber out unaided. I can then provide her with a coffee, a tasty and challengingly large muffin (no poppy seeds) and a magazine with pictures of kittens in; and sit down myself for at least an hour. Sometimes I get to read a book. Ben can come too, there are special hidey holes for the kids to read in, buttons to press for spoken stories, computers and more comfy sofas. Whole families spend their Sundays there. It's full of the sort of beautiful people who have even tans and suit their shorts. It's the place to be and be seen and it's a book shop. I love this country.

* * *

I said tomato today. And it rhymed with potato. I am distraught. It's the beginning of the end of my English accent and therefore my instant access to friends and popularity. The trouble is, it's hard to say 'no tomato thank you' any other way to a busy server in *Harvey's*. They mishear you if you're not careful and I don't like tomato, whatever it rhymes with. *Harvey's* by the way is the most delightful fast-food chain ever. (I know you think delightful fast food an oxymoron but you haven't been to *Harvey's*.) They construct atop your chosen burger, before your very eyes, beautiful little montages of any selection of umpteen garnishes you care to list with the most affectionate care I've seen since my mother prepared me meals with faces on. In fact, I reckon that if you asked for a face made of lettuce and olive slices and one strip of hot pepper for the mouth they'd be glad to oblige. I'd better not try it though, Ben gets embarrassed enough in places where I am able to ask for Buffalo Wings.

The great tomato debacle punctuated a long-awaited and much appreciated weekend off. Several of the carers who helped Pat through the time before I arrived here have fallen by the wayside for one reason or another (not all to do with muddy pebbles) and the next few to appear on an experimental basis haven't all been able to handle Zuscha the way Pat would like; but we now have two special ladies who are willing and able to suspend normality for a while in the interests of keeping me sane. It's about time I introduced them to you.

Mary comes from the Red Cross twice a week for three hours and is my source of evenings out. She loves the way I pronounce things, likes Zuscha enough to tolerate the mess and is not fazed by phone calls from strange gentlemen. She wishes to vet Computer Hero shortly and make sure he is good enough for me. She'd hate for a Canadian to let me down.

Holly is my weekend-off fairy and has made it her mission in life to work with elderly people. She sees it as the only growth industry left and wishes to be the best there is. She is. Holly really is good for Zuscha whereas I play at it when I'm not too tired. They sing, they dance, they pore over old photos, they chat. When Holly has been in charge Zuscha glows with happiness. Pat trusts Holly to cope overnight. I wondered why, with such talent in town, Pat had settled for me. 'I turned the job down' Holly told me, 'I couldn't handle it 24/7.'

It was Holly therefore who arrived on Friday evening so that Ben and I could spend the weekend camping with Computer Hero and co. It sounded great, sleeping under the stars, fishing to keep the kids happy, beer for the grown-ups, mayhap a spot of canoeing. We would learn all about the great outdoors and become a little more Canadian. It sounded great and we couldn't wait to get going. I rang as soon as we were ready to escape to say we were on our way.

'Where shall we meet you?'

'What for?'

'The camping trip, shall we go straight to Elora or pick you up on the way?

'Camping?'

'Did you forget?'

'Forget what?'

I am no longer in love. Mary will not be pleased.

We were left with a long weekend to fill, no intention of staying at home and no time to plan any touring, so we jumped in the car to see where we ended up.

Where we ended up was in a town called Hamilton, not far from Toronto. Hardly a tourist destination, it's a steel town sited on Lake Ontario and thus boasts an interesting mix of industrial history and tolerable beaches. It would do at a pinch. Surprisingly enough, Hamilton turned out to be remarkably well stocked with museums. Ben loves museums. (I don't know why, I hated them as a kid. Still do.) So we managed to make the most of our weekend of freedom despite its non-camping nature. The Children's Museum had an interactive dinosaur display (no I don't know how you interact with a dinosaur, ask Ben) and the Steam and Technology Museum was in the throes of its 16th

Annual Antique Steam and Gas Engine Show. This was a hoot. I quote from the brochure:

> *This event showcases the work of dedicated individuals who collect and operate antique engines or build models of the steam and gas engines of the past. The exhibitors, volunteers and museum staff will happily answer your questions.*

They will not however happily let you play with their trains. Each little scale model had a little seat on top for its driver. Each little seat had room for two, a bit like a motor bike. Each little scale model with seats for two ran round the exhibition site with one or two grown adults on it, followed by a sprinkling of small boys who couldn't work out why it wasn't their turn yet. I generally try not to influence Ben with my occasionally irritable incomprehension of the male of the species. I know it's not healthy for a small boy to hear such things at an impressionable age but eventually the only explanation I could reasonably supply for this phenomenon was that grown men aren't as good as children at sharing their toys.

Hamilton also boasts a traffic roundabout (I think it's the only one in the country. I certainly haven't come across one before, going round it in the wrong direction felt very strange) and lots more big sky. Have I mentioned the sky yet? I really should have done by now, it's strange how the most enormous difference of all is so pervasive that it goes without saying. You can see the sky here. And it's huge. I sort of noticed when we first arrived, enjoyed being dwarfed by it and started to clock the different clouds but it was only when we popped home that I realised we don't have sky in England. Well, we do but you have to look up to see it so you don't really bother. When there's a little square atop a tube of buildings it doesn't shout at you. Here the sky screams 'Hi, aren't I big and gorgeous?' every time you pop your head outside. When we came back from our wedding expedition I realised it was mainly the sky I'd been missing. I made two resolutions on the spot. One was to learn to look upwards all the time and the other was never again to live somewhere where you had to.

Zuscha and Holly survived their weekend extremely well, although Holly apparently had a terrifying encounter with Ben's *Wallace and Gromit* alarm clock. She just wasn't expecting to hear 'Morning Gromit, time for walkies!' first thing in the morning and completely failed to associate the Yorkshire accent with a plasticene film character. She hunted high and low for the intruder before inflicting serious but not terminal damage on the clock. Zuscha fared better, only going to the bus stop twice, which is average for when Pat leaves to be replaced by me. Pat and I seem to be interchangeable now, which was the original plan, so I am brimming with renewed confidence in my ability to cope. Not so confident in my newfound role as transatlantic femme fatale however. Some things never change.

The cats had grapes in their bowl this morning.

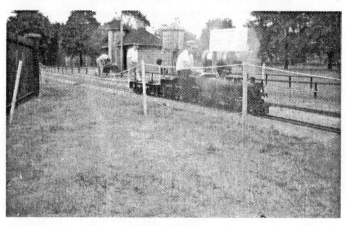

Big boys' toys

EIGHT

The Big One

Big news. *The K/W Record*, my source of all information – CNN doesn't count, at least *The Record* is supposed to be parochial – has a world news page, from which I occasionally learn what is happening of significance in England. This week I read that a slate has been unearthed in Tintagel which might bear an inscription a bit like the Latin version of a name similar to Arthur. I also read that it 'adds a new dimension to the debate about the possibility of there having been a real Arthur on whom the mythical figure was based.' No it doesn't, it could equally well just mean that a Latin version of a name similar Arthur was popular back then, but that's not the point. I have clearly misunderstood the concept of world news until now. This could be the page to watch.

Even bigger news. *The Record* reports a new category of profession eligible for immigration. Exotic dancers may enter the country now, because Canadian girls won't strip any more. *The Record* is incredulous, so clearly I am not the only one who finds this faintly bizarre. As a sort-of English version of a paramedic with out-of-date qualifications, a Master's degree in Psychology and a City and Guilds in cake decorating, I am a dangerous foreign worker who has to be watched very carefully in case I steal a job from a Canadian. I must promise to leave the country the moment my visa expires. If I were a stripper however, my landed immigrant status would be assured. Not any old stripper I should add, one has to be able to prove one's professional status. A delightful editorial in *The Record* wonders just how the poor overworked immigration official will be able to verify one's authenticity. Apparently a portfolio of photographs is likely to be sufficient, which is rather disappointing. I'd love to be able to imagine the interviews, 'and exactly how exotic is your dancing Ma'am?' Maybe I could just flash my tattoo and hope for the best.

Meanwhile Zuscha is making the life of a live-in carer pretty exotic. She has got stuck under the garden fence twice this week. Her joints are stiffening up quite rapidly – which is allowable when you are 77 – but in her version of the world she's as agile as ever. The obvious answer to spying a particularly tantalizing weed in next door's garden is to take the most direct route. Getting her out is a tricky business as of the two of us I'm the only one who knows she's stuck. I tried dismantling the fence permanently so that she can just walk through – our long-suffering neighbours have no prize possessions left along that side of their house, Zuscha's already had them all – but this has made her cross. Maybe it doesn't present enough of a challenge. Or possibly she remembers that there should be a fence there, either way she has spent many a happy hour rebuilding it. She can get stuck nicely again now, in the sun, just as the weather hots up for real.

The summer holidays are in full swing and Ben has gone to Camp. Proper camping Camp, where they stay overnight and light fires and do healthy outdoor stuff. I am distraught.

As I waved him off on the bus with his little sleeping bag all rolled up and his big bag of bug repellent and wasp sting cream, I welled up with tears and sobbed all the way home. It was like having a temporary amputation. Travel hasn't done anything healthy for my separation anxiety and life on Planet Alzheimer is seriously damaging to one's sense of proportion. I think I am becoming a little neurotic. As soon as I had dried my eyes it occurred to me that all I'd done the previous week was shout at him for being under my feet all day. I was off blubbing again. He knew I was only shouting at him because I couldn't shout at Zuscha and that I was only shouting at anybody because I wasn't in love any more. He kept saying 'It's all right Mummy, I understand.' I am guilty and miserable and a terrible mother again and I almost want to go home.

There was nothing for it but to forgive Computer Hero and go back to doing all that dopey stuff that successful modern women with tattoos don't do, especially the travelling sort who thought they were too clever to sit by the telephone. Mary and Holly are naturally as up-to-date with developments as I am, in fact there are days when they predict the unreliable memory better than I do. They disapprove mightily and think that I should demand better treatment from a beau. And of course I should. I know that. I'm kidding myself he can't help it because, pathetic though it may sound, I need something to do with my time off. In which case, who's using who? I'm just not used to conducting a not-quite-relationship in quite such a glare of publicity. There's something pretty demeaning about having to ring and ask someone to let you out to play. And then ringing back and telling them not to bother because you've been forgotten. And then ringing back and …maybe I should just grow up.

By the time Ben came home from camp I had pulled myself together enough to be planning a spot of gentle sightseeing. I went to meet the bus eager to discuss where we should go next but Ben wasn't there. I spent a worrisome half hour scouring the faces of the kids as they emerged and began to think I'd met the wrong bus. In the end there was only one kid left, sitting despondently but patiently on the grass. He was about a foot taller than the Ben I remembered from last week and wore a huge new fishing hat. He forgave me in the end. He has been sailing and fishing, singing and investigating beaver dams. I am delighted to have him home and keep on insisting on hugs. That's horrible when you're nine.

We sightsaw next quite nearby in the Mennonite village of St. Jacobs. Much of southern Ontario is farmed by Mennonites, who crossed the Pond at about the same time as the Amish people who settled in the States. Both are groups of Anabaptists who were persecuted out of Europe, they are just descended from different families. If I have understood the St Jacobs multi-media presentation correctly (of which more shortly) Anabaptists are simply people who choose to baptise their followers as adults rather than babies and have opted for a simple lifestyle. I can't see the problem with this myself but then Europe does tend to gang up on minorities every generation or so. My forebears, being Jewish, ended up in England in my great-grandfather's time for similar reasons.

The Mennonites wear a distinctively traditional costume and the stricter orders travel in horse-drawn buggies, machinery in all its forms being forbidden. All our local roads have extra wide hard shoulders to accommodate the buggies without inconveniencing other traffic. There's even a special triangular warning road sign, a black horse drawn buggy on a yellow background of course. There seem to be a lot of different levels of simplicity and some families allow themselves farm machinery and telephones. A few have taken to cars but only if all the chrome is blacked out.

This means that the car is purely utilitarian rather than for show. My level of empathy dips alarmingly about here.

I had avoided the inevitable trip to St. Jacobs (*the Heart of Mennonite Country*) itself for quite a long while. It's the place for hand stitched quilts and home made pies and you can watch traditional crafts in action, the blacksmith, the weaver and the broom-maker. I don't know how I feel about a people turning themselves into a side-show. Strangely enough I could deal with Niagara having become a money machine without too much trouble. I'm not sure about the same happening to a religious community.

The village is delightful to look at. The buildings are quaint, the church meeting houses beautiful and the craft shops plentiful. Recorded hymns sing out from amplifiers on the church roof and echo up and down the little main street. It's as pretty as any chocolate box Little-Something-on-the-Water in Wiltshire, such a cute place that it can't help making a killing by sending itself up. Occasionally there's a reminder of the real life behind the tweeness. A covered 'buggy park' next to the meeting house, an old order Mennonite gentleman selling maple syrup from his buggy by the roadside, girls in demure gauze bonnets behind the counters. But mainly there's the kitsch and the coachloads of American and Japanese tourists lapping it up.

We began with the blacksmith, Ben is contemplating lessons. We toured the shops and I had a few moments of wondering what happened to the enormous amount of revenue dropping from the pockets of the herds of well-heeled visitors being corralled from gift shop to quilt emporium to Information Centre, containing multi-media presentation. But then we visited the aforementioned multiple media and I learned that my cynicism was probably misplaced. The families live by their industries, farming and marketing of home produced goodies. Did you know most real maple syrup is made by Mennonites because it's so labour intensive? The revenue from quilts and tourism funds a huge disaster relief project which sends teams of Mennonites from their homes to help out in trouble spots around the world. (Presumably it's OK to use machinery in a crisis.)

The presentation is fascinating by the way. Beautifully laid out, well organised and free, although donations are happily accepted by a quietly charming chappie who makes your average Canadian seem a little brusque. I think I was expecting a rather dour lecture on the perils of modern living but by film and pictures, models and voice-overs I was introduced to a quiet, happy and family-orientated community who love their food and will happily bake as many pies as visitors to their farmers' market wish to buy. Sadly, judging by the relative crowdedness of the Information Centre and the Christmas decoration store, education seems to be beneath the notice of most serious professional shoppers so presumably many of St Jacobs' visitors miss the chance to get the point.

I was charmed enough to consider buying a quilt. When I get back I might want a souvenir of Mennonite Country. Mind you if I wanted a patchwork quilt in my home badly enough I probably would have made one myself by now. I can sew too. Maybe I won't.

* * *

Zuscha opened the car door while we were going along today. Frightened out of my wits, I shouted at her. She was terribly crestfallen. In an effort to try and cheer us up I took her out for French fries. Big treat. She dipped them in her coffee of course. Always does. We did all our favourite things, we looked at the kittens in the pet shop and agreed they were good doggies, we read all the signs over all the shops out loud, having a good giggle about the *Superior Memorials*. We shared our best joke – Zuscha sees something faintly surprising and says 'Sheesh!' I then have to say 'Sheesh kebab!' Zuscha has to reply 'At least!' And then we laugh. I don't know why.

And then, out of nowhere the big crisis hit. There had been warnings enough and I probably should have seen it coming but I didn't. Got totally pissed off with men, got totally pissed off with Zuscha, got totally pissed off with Ben, burst into tears and wanted to catch the next flight home. All of a sudden it was all too much. I didn't want to spend the foreseeable future yelling at a deaf old lady to PUT THE PAPER IN THE TOILET ten times a day, cooking meals that are forgotten the second they're eaten, burbling about kebabs and doggies all day, babysitting for the entire street because I'm always there and being messed around and taken for granted by a man with a normal life to live. I wanted out. Now. Adventures aren't fun, they're hard and stressful and they make you cry. I wanted my bed, my rules and my sanity back. I wanted to sleep for a week, cry for another week and then sleep some more. Somewhere unmuddy.

Everyone rallied round to help me through it. Well, except the man obviously. All my respite carers offered to work extra shifts, even the exes. Some invited us to their homes as well – while the others took their turns with Zuschy – for dinner, or a chat or a sleep, whatever I needed to let off steam in peace and try to relax. I am extremely grateful and rather humbled. These ladies don't have to be my friends, they get paid to Zuscha-sit. With more moral support than I had any right to expect (and several new friends) the Big One eased off into the background. It didn't quite go away, it hung around the edges, waving from time to time, like those kids who can't resist jumping up and down at the back of a crowd when it's being televised.

The Big One left me with a need to know where it had come from, analysis essential to head off another attack before I really did book those flights. Ben was having far too much fun and would never forgive me now. I had a feeling that excessive introspection was probably unhealthy but naval-gazing is a hard habit to break when the alternative topics of the day have to do with birdies in trees and toilet paper.

What happened? Was it just the wounded ego of a daft middle-aged woman who thinks she's sixteen again because she's met some bloke who doesn't object to passing the time of day over a beer? Was it just lack of sleep? A combination of the two? Or something more to do with the travelling lark being harder than I'd supposed? I came to the conclusion that, sleep and stupidity notwithstanding, it was probably partly to do with the transition between extended holiday and real life. The novelty suddenly wore off and reality set in with a vengeance. It was like hitting a brick wall. What do marathon runners call that bit where you either quit or finish? Must find out, if that was my version of it then maybe Ben is safe from any more nonsense.

Feeling better now though. Named, analysed and tamed, the Big One is still waving intermittently from the back of the crowd but it has stopped leaping about with a banner that says 'Hello Mum!' I may be single again but at least I've got my sense of humour back.

And only just in time, otherwise I might have missed out on some more vitally important World News. *Experts baffled by 'near-mess' over Windsor*. Would you believe it? Some poo escaped from an aeroplane and landed in Windsor while the Queen was at home. It's OK though because a Buckingham Palace spokesman said the Queen was not aware of the incident. Still wondering about the real world. Must buy a short wave radio and try to find the World Service, I'm starting to miss the Beeb.

I took Ben out for dinner to make up for being a ratty, neurotic, bad-tempered, tearful apology for a parent. We decided to try *East Side Mario's* 'exciting Italian American cuisine'. Incidentally I've never understood how any cooking other than French can be 'cuisine' but that's beside the point. It was indeed most exciting, waiters breaking into four-part harmony in honour of someone's birthday etc. The cuisine was definitely Italian (pasta) and American (enormous) and I found myself once again overawed by a culture that feels comfortable worshipping its food.

I am getting used to the 'all you can eat' yardstick for portion sizes and no longer apologise for asking to have things the way I want them but am now au-fait with a new way to adore the stuff on your plate. Each server in *East Side Mario's* carries, clipped to his or her belt, a little viewer like the ones you can buy at any seaside town. You know the sort of thing, binoculars with a circular set of slides fitted in, so you can hold them up to the light and squint at a selection of sea views. Only these aren't sea views. These are the desserts.

Yes, once you have read the mouth-watering details of your towering triple chocolate thingamajig with extra whatnots, you can inspect a photograph to ensure that it actually does tower enough. OK I know we put our desserts on a trolley. It serves the same purpose but we Brits still get away with the idea that we don't really want to eat it. We point and say 'oh all right I'll have some of that then'. Here, by the time you've read the description, borrowed the viewer, scanned through to find and inspect your chosen confection and ordered it by name, there's no way to pretend you're just eating it to be polite. I didn't realise we felt so guilty about our food until I lived with people who don't.

I'm reminded of a story one of our early respite ladies told me about her daughter's visit to England. She went into a pub for lunch and ordered a ham and cheese sandwich. But she couldn't have a ham and cheese sandwich. She could have a ham sandwich. Or a cheese sandwich. That's what it said on the menu for goodness sake. Obviously she ordered one of each, deconstructed them at the table and ended up with exactly what she wanted. I'm not that brave yet, although I have finally plucked up the courage to request my salad without croutons and bacon bits. It has taken me months to get this far and do you know what? The sky doesn't fall in and nobody shouts at you. If you only want salad items in your salad it's allowed. Bizarre.

The waitress who has adopted us in *Gatto's* (the best veggie burgers in town and sauerkraut to die for) looked at me a little strangely the first time I tried it. Asking for my salad without bits.

'That's fine but you always had them before.'

'I didn't know I was allowed to ask you to leave them out.'

This is the lady who fetches me tiny little samples of menu items I can't identify from the name to try; and who can remember from visit to visit that Zuscha's smoked meat sandwich had to come with brown bread instead of rye (easier on the dentures) on a big plate (less messy) with a knife and fork (it's a bit too big to be recognisable as a sandwich) and without the cocktail stick holding it together (tends to get eaten). She deserves for me to have asked her name. I'm sorry.

* * *

In an effort to settle down a little more reliably I finally did go out and buy that short wave radio. 'Reintroduce the Beeb to your life' I thought, 'a spot of British sanity for those difficult days.' I was really looking forward to regular fixes of the World Service but finding it seems to be a full time hobby. I read a book by Terry Waite some years ago about his time as a hostage in Beirut. I recall reading how the World Service filled their days and I now realise that he is equally likely to have meant finding it as listening to it.

The Beeb kindly emailed the correct frequencies to me. There are eight to choose from for North America (Eastern and Central). Each operates at a different time of day and the times are given as GMT. I know that on this side of Canada we are five hours behind the UK but it's summer, so is that four hours behind GMT or six? One can miss a whole programme doing the conversion. I've constructed a little chart to speed that bit up but then there's walking round the house waggling the aerial about to find the point of least interference for that time of day. Sometimes there are two frequencies going at once, reception for each being best in a different part of the house – or possibly garden. By the time I've darted to and fro comparing sound quality (absence of) the programme is over. I can hear best, predictably enough, during *Sports Roundup* and an odd soap called *Westway* which appears to be about a doctor's surgery under the A40 flyover where I'm sure there was a travellers' settlement when I used to drive ambulances around Paddington. It isn't a patch on *The Archers*.

From radio to TV now and we have made our British television debut. Part one of our episode of *Moving People* – up to the moment of closing our front door in London – was broadcast this week, part two follows next Thursday. Yes, John Peel has introduced us, well mainly Ben, to the nation. We are nearly famous. If you count Channel 4.

Fortunately we have no way of seeing it here so I can pretend it's not real. I have had to rely on friendly emailers to tell me all about it and reassure me that I didn't have spinach in my teeth or anything. With thirteen hours of rushes to choose from and eight minutes to fill, one or two bits didn't make it, the magic show for example. After all that angst. They did however opt to keep in an unwise mention in an unguarded moment of my recently acquired tattoo. This will come as a bit of a surprise to the Mumster. I wonder how she'll react to hearing about it from a TV programme?

Tattoo-related awkwardness aside, all comments have been complimentary so far. I've received emails from complete strangers who enjoyed it and think we're terribly brave and stuff, which is somewhat embarrassing after my recent tantrum. Ben has captured the hearts of the British viewing public, which bodes well for him earning his keep as a TV star when we return penniless from our adventure, possibly sooner rather than later.

It's nearing the end of the summer holidays and we have a week off coming up. I have maps and tour guides spread liberally around the floor in my room and am trying to work out how much of Ontario we can 'do' in a week. I still find it impossible to estimate journey times. The distances are so enormous that I have no conception of how far it is from a to b. Knowing it's further than I can comprehend, I assume it will take days to drive there. I can't yet add in to the equation the fact that there are no cars in between. No traffic jams, roundabouts, contraflows, gyratory systems or 'ring-of-steel' City Police roadblocks. Just straight, empty roads. It might be a long way but once you've started you keep on driving, so actually it's not so far after all.

Trying to work out how long it will take to get somewhere here puts me in mind of those optical illusions you learn about in undergraduate psychology lectures, where two lines don't look the same length but are. I know it takes an hour to get from Kitchener to Toronto, which is another city, and I know it takes an hour to get from Harringay to Edgware, which are both Greater London, but the ideas seem wrong side by side.

My first blueprint itinerary is almost ready for inspection by people who know the place. It involves a round trip taking in Ottawa, the Algonquin National Park and some terribly old rock carvings. Oh and a beaver dam or two and the highest canal lock in the world and some reconstructed native villages. If it can be done in a week I'll treat myself to a doughnut.

NINE

Lakes and flagpoles

We never did get to Ottawa. Our week off evaporated into two days and there wasn't time to go that far. A slight hitch on the 'buying a lump of land to build a house on' front meant that Pat couldn't come back from BC to cover for me without leaving negotiations at a critical stage. This has been happening rather a lot lately, there always seems to be something to make my time off impossibly inconvenient. Pat assures me that we will be able to reclaim all my lost days once we move and I am sure she is right but just for once, I would like to make a plan that works out.

I managed to talk Holly into staying here for a couple of nights so we could still celebrate the last week of the hols in style but we reined in our ambitions a little.

We headed north, to Georgian Bay. This is a sort of nose attached to Lake Huron – if you imagine it as a face looking westwards – and boasts the world's longest freshwater beach, thirty thousand islands (gosh) and plenty of historical thingies to nose around feeling educational.

We gave the beach a miss. I've always found trips to sand and water depressing. There's something about a beach full of proper families with Dads and everything that points out that there are only two of us with devastating cruelty, so we began with a slight detour to Blue Mountain instead. Ostensibly to visit the Scenic Caves but also to try out the go-kart run down said mountain side. In the winter the area is a ski resort and someone hit on the idea of making money from the incline all year round by transporting lunatics like us to the top on a ski lift and then allowing us to hurtle down 1,600 feet on a little toboggan-type thing in a zig-zaggy gully, reminiscent of a concrete bobsleigh track.

Terrifying. And such fun that we made another detour on the way home to do it again. The caves were pretty spectacular too. I've never seen Maidenhair Ferns growing wild before. Well, to be honest I've never seen one grow at all, they just die in my bathroom. We finally fetched up at *Saint Marie among the Hurons*, a reconstructed Jesuit Mission in Midland which was established in the1600s to convert the local native people to Catholicism. It all went horribly wrong in the end of course and everybody died. *The Martyrs' Shrine* is just over the road. No-one else seems to be struck by the irony of this.

Historical sites have changed a bit since my childhood. There are 'costumed interpreters' lurking round every corner, showing you what might have been happening at the time. If I'd read about them before we went I'd have gone all sniffy about dumbing down but I'm now a total convert, completely charmed by these efforts to recreate the past for me. It may sound pathetic but I'm not much of a historian and it comes alive for me too when you walk into the kitchen and someone is making corn bread on the stove.

We found a healthy dose of candour too, there's a genuine concern to explain that people can honestly have what they misguidedly believe to be good intentions and still precipitate a total disaster. This is particularly true of the Mission of Saint Marie; which started as a humanitarian effort to bring medicine and the gospel to the Huron and ended with the native people (whose need for either is pretty debatable) being decimated by a combination of internal division between those who converted and those who did not; and the introduction of new European diseases to which they had no resistance. I came away feeling that they'd been pretty fair to everyone and Ben came away with some complicated ideas to discuss ad infinitum in the car on the next leg of the journey. Things can be wrong even if nobody means to be bad for example, and thinking you know what's good for someone else isn't always very clever. There are times when I think that my patronising and conceited excuses to his English schoolteachers about travelling being a living education weren't so wide of the mark.

We had to cruise round the thirty thousand islands of course. And that's a whole lot of islands, although sadly I can't tell you who it was who first counted them all. Some of them are pretty small – just like the cartoon desert island, a bit of rock and a single tree – but many are just big enough for a solitary house. And a flagpole. Canadians sure do love their flag, it's everywhere. Not just on civic buildings and in parks but outside ordinary houses. In fact there's a bungalow in Kitchener with the Maple Leaf design picked out in red tiles on the roof. I didn't realise quite how odd I found this until I saw a flag outside each solitary house on each little island just big enough to put a house on among the thirty thousand islands of Georgian Bay. Any such unleashing of the Union Jack is viewed rather dimly by the English chattering classes, a suspicious and unwelcome dose of patriotism in a country that oughtn't to be proud of itself. The cross of St George is even more suspect with all manner of reactionary overtones. I suppose Canada's national pride comes without a side order of guilt.

Zuscha was glad to see us when we came back. During one of her regular conversations with Misha The Smaller she pointed to me and said, 'Oh yes, she looks after me you know.' I wasn't sure whether to be pleased that she realised I didn't bug her all day just for the hell of it, or sad that she has realised she needs looking after.

* * *

With the summer holidays finally over, Ben is back at school. It's been a long haul. The school break is ten weeks long for goodness sake. That's almost twice as long as we're used to. Apparently this dates back to when children were needed for farm work and nobody's got around to asking whether it's still sensible. There are no half term breaks, so the kids will work solidly through the year now apart from two weeks at Christmas and a week in March. I'm not sure that I like this at all. I know that British working mums complain about half terms, I certainly did but I have a feeling that the academic year here will get pretty exhausting. Then they can forget all they've learned again next summer.

I miscalculated quite badly on the summer camp front. I booked Ben into three schemes in all, two of which were just day camps, not wanting to be 'sending him away' all the time after the upheaval of moving. I also wanted to make the most of being a stay-at-home Mum for once, it's never happened before. All the other parents, wised up to ten week summers, had their kids booked into camps solidly week after week so there has been nobody around for him to play with. He's been a bit bored and I've been responsible. I am at a loss to understand how we could adjust to so much so fast and completely miss the point when it came to something as simple as a longer school holiday. I'll know better next year.

It has done him good to be in school at the start of things this term. He's busy volunteering for everything in sight and, although he'd be the first to say that he enjoyed feeling special last term, I get the impression he's even happier to be normal this time round. With that in mind I'm considering approaching Pat with the idea of co-ordinating our move with the start of a term. She will be back here soon, yes really this time, as the land for our new house has been finalised (hooray, you can see the sea from it) so I'll broach the subject then and see if it's an acceptable suggestion.

One of the jobs Ben's volunteered for is Safety Patrol. This means teams of older kids donning reflective jackets and manning the road junctions outside school, seeing everyone safely across. The London parent in me freaked at the very idea but it sunk in eventually that there's no traffic to speak of outside Prueter Public School – apart from parents who know that the kids are their marshals – therefore having children do this is a relatively safe exercise in early responsibility. I'm pleased, with an eye to future CVs, that he's taking on extra-curriculars but have to confess to a moment of miffedness when I realised we'd have to be up and about earlier in the morning every other week.

Zuscha isn't sleeping you see. So neither am I. Again. There have always been several nights in a week when she's up and about but this is getting ridiculous. I'm calling it a good night when I only get up three times. In desperation I've started giving her Melatonin before bed. This is yet another herbal marvel I'd not heard of before, a hormone that is supposed to help your body recognise that it needs to wind down at night-time. I have discovered its benefits somewhat belatedly, according to Pat she was taking it for a while before we arrived but had it stopped by some visiting respite nurse because it made Zuscha go and get the bus one night and was therefore a Bad Thing. I wish I'd known about that little episode months ago. Zuscha goes to get the bus when she's looking for someone and when she's cross.

Anyway, the nights have calmed down somewhat. She still gets up several times but seems more aware that it's night time. She creeps about now and ends up back in bed eventually, as opposed to the all-singing all-dancing knickers-on-the-lampshades sort of nights we were getting used to. (Don't ask.)

As I write this, Zuscha is dunking an apple cinnamon biscuit in her gravy. It must be nice, there goes another.

The odd snatches of sleep are helping my hay fever a bit but not much. I used to get slight hay fever at home. Nothing too unpleasant, the odd snuffle, itchy eyes, I always put it down to the pollution and congratulated myself on being free of such irritations now we live somewhere clean. And I was, until the second week in September. Suddenly I've been hit with an allergy so violent I spent two days convinced it was flu. The clever money is on Ragweed and the homeopathic thingies I brought with me from home aren't a match for it at all. Off to the drugstore for a fraught attempt to work out, with the aid of a long-suffering pharmacist, what they call things over here that may or may not be the same as the things over there that make me sicker than the hay fever does.

On the up side, I sounded so ill on the phone that Pat has decided to come and give us that break. It looks as though we'll end up with about five days away so the maps are all over the floor again. We can't decide whether to resurrect the Ottawa tour or to go for somewhere different now the weather is less predictable. The parks we had planned on stopping in to break the journey could be pretty miserable if it rains, so we're tempted to strike out north again instead of east. It's time for autumn trees and that's where they're best so I'm told.

The current top destination is Tobermory. I didn't know everyone's favourite womble was named after a place in Canada until I scrutinised a map of Ontario, embarrassing really. From there we can get a glass-bottomed boat out into Lake Huron and look for shipwrecks. We can also catch the ferry to Manitoulin Island, where they've found the earliest signs of human habitation in the whole of Canada. Ben likes such facts. Did you know that Manitoulin Island is the largest island in an inland lake in the world?

While waiting to be set free there's plenty in K/W to keep us amused. We went to the Waterloo Medieval Festival on Sunday. It was organised by the same guy who ran the Waterloo Busker Carnival a few weeks ago. He seems to organise everything come to think of it. I'm not used to local extravaganzas, unless you count the Notting Hill Carnival, which isn't quite the same thing as I won't attend that for less than ten pounds an hour on emergency standby. It took a while to get into the spirit of things. My first impression of the Busker Carnival, *an annual international celebration of street theatre*, was that you could see better in Covent Garden any weekend of the year. As I wandered about though, watching the performers carefully making a fuss of as many kids as they could, I began to understand how truly community oriented these events are. The main street was out of action for almost a week for the construction of stages. No-one moaned. All the shops and businesses sponsored something. There was a big concert for the kids, as well as one for adults and a final family bash, after which dancing in the street was compulsory. One or two of the acts weren't bad but hey who needs talent as long as everyone gets involved?

The Medieval effort was similarly naff but we all turned out and put our hands in our pockets anyway. I've never lived in a small town before, so my cultural snobbery is probably a little misplaced. It was all very nice. Just a bit, well, unsophisticated. And I'm starting to realise that that doesn't really matter at all.

* * *

Thanks to Pat we got to Tobermory in the end. Followed by Manitoulin Island and Parry Sound. In between, a lot of lakes and a whole bunch of trees. I am finally starting to understand immenseness – yes I know it's a big place, the biggest individual country in the world, we absorbed such information while planning the move – but there are different sorts of big. We didn't drive far really, it was just a long way.

Did you know Ontario has a quarter of a million lakes? That's another snippet I absorbed during the research phase, I am realising what that means too. The place is like a honeycomb. When the first few lakes hove into view we stopped and got out of the car to say things like 'isn't it lovely?' and take a photo. Then the penny dropped. There's another lake round every corner, and another, and another, and they are all uniformly scenic. Then there are more lakes. One photo entitled 'general lakeness' will suffice and what's more, eventually you don't want to see a lake round the next corner because it just means you have to detour round it to get where you're going.

Tobermory is pretty. And little. Faintly English in fact, an attractive harbour with arty little shops and no food chains or shopping malls. Sadly our shipwreck spotting trip was curtailed due to a 'tornado watch' involving the sort of thunder storm that deprives people of their power supply and produces 'hailstones the size of gumballs' as Ben subsequently informed everyone. Nothing so puny as rain. Even the weather is bigger here. We saw one or two wrecks from our glass-bottomed boat before the storm rolled in. Ben was most excited but I found the whole thing rather sad in the end. One minute you're bobbing along on the surface doing what you've got to do and the next, nothing but petrified remains. Then people come and gawp. It put me in mind of my marriage a bit.

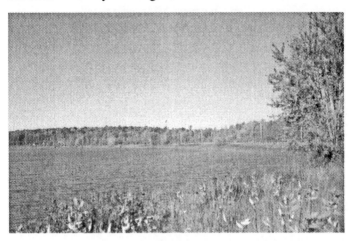

General lakeness

The ferry to Manitoulin taught me more about bigness. Two hours on a car ferry out of sight of land to get to… another bit of Ontario. Not even another province, let alone another country. Kept saying 'it's a lake' to myself, quietly of course, trying to make the idea sink in but it wouldn't. How can you possibly be inland when you can't see the horizon? It's a kind of perceptual travel sickness.

It's not just the space that makes me dizzy, it's the emptiness too. Canada has approximately six people per square mile and we come from a country with a population density of about 220. As most of each Canadian six are huddled near the US border that leaves very few people to bump into further north. Somewhere, miles from the next nearest human being, in the middle of the biggest island in an inland lake in the world I had a panic attack. It all started when we drove down a deserted lane that looked really pretty, just to see where it went. It went a long way, that's where it went. Past dense woodland and signs saying

'Do not enter – bears' and the like. Eventually, several kilometres from the (deserted) main road, the (deserted) track petered out and became a (deserted) lake. Ben went pebble hunting. I fell apart. Nobody knew where we were. Nobody knew who we were. Suppose he fell in, suppose the car wouldn't start, suppose…well anything unforeseen really. How long would we last? How far could we walk? How far could I carry him? I finally twigged that this lump of land deserves and probably often demands a little more respect than I had hitherto given it. At least a first aid kit in the car, some emergency rations and a blanket maybe. I had my trusty AA card with me but it wouldn't have been much use, we'd have resorted to eating it before managing to locate a telephone.

People regularly tell me horrifying tales of going fishing and spending three days trying to find their car again and I put Ben in our less than reliable heap with no more than a bag of crisps and a bottle of Coke. Felt irresponsible again and frightened and stupid and too overwrought to admire some truly stupendous pebbles. And to realise that I was looking at the biggest lake in an island in an inland lake in the world.

Moving swiftly on, we finally found a little place with houses, not exactly a town or a village, probably best described as a community. It had a sort of restaurant and a sort of B&B, so we survived the night in the tender care of a nice lady who rents out her daughter's room now she has left home. We both seem to bring out maternal instincts in the people we meet these days, I must look a little overwrought. Some TLC and, later on, a huge plate of pasta restored my adventurous spirit. TLC and pasta generally do. Determined to turn over a new leaf I carefully packed the leftovers in a cool-box for emergencies; said a lot of heartfelt thank-yous for our comfortable and comforting night and turned my attention to the next leg of our journey. Heading home we planned to pick up the Trans-Canada Highway for a short way and then turn south around the side of Georgian Bay, ovenighting in Parry Sound, a town that looked half way home.

The Trans-Canada Highway was less exciting that it sounded, just a long straight road really. What was I expecting you ask in superior tones? Dunno really, it just sounded romantic. That part of the journey would almost have been boring if it hadn't been for the strange mystery of the Parry Sound trains. This odd little town was indeed about half way home. Not much to see, it's a harbour with a nice little museum and a lookout tower that used to be for fire watching although only peculiar tourists like us climb it now. There's also a railway bridge. A huge, enormously high railway bridge with girders and stuff that dominates the otherwise pretty skyline from every point of the compass. It's so awful it's almost beautiful. I took an arty photo looking up from underneath it in a vain attempt to be a proper photographer.

Trains ran constantly, we heard train-type whistling noises Doppler shifting their way past our motel room window quite late into the night *but no trains ever went over that bridge*. I kept leaping to the window to check. Where did they come from? Where did they go? Did they exist or were they the ghostly auditory remains of trains long since passed? Spooky.

The pasta wasn't so nice when we got home. Which was a shame, it might have made a handy and nutritious late night snack. I'm losing weight you see. This is odd on a diet of doughnuts and beer. It must be a combination of running after Zuscha all day and going off chocolate. Last time I went off chocolate I was pregnant but I think the cause is a little less alarming this time, it's just too sweet.

There is too much sugar in everything. Even the savoury stuff. I've learned the hard way to check labels very carefully, sweetened mayonnaise was a horrible shock I can tell you. There's sugar in peanut butter, pasta sauce, even the flax seed bread Pat likes us to get from the health food store is sweetened with honey. They'd sweeten the eggs if they could. As for the chocolate, you might as well be eating sugar lumps. I thought I'd be clever and buy brands from home – Cadbury's and the like – but most of it's manufactured over here to a different recipe, a special transatlantic, extra sugar recipe. It's extremely nasty.

The reason for all this sugar? They take all the fat out of everything to make it good for you. Once all the fat has gone, you need to add sugar to make things taste right. People want fat-free products because everybody has a weight problem. But then, if they didn't put sugar in everything…

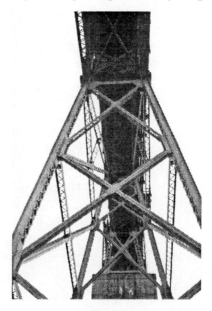

Spooky

TEN

Pumpkin people and leaf hoovers

Back in K/W the teachers are on strike. It's rather fun. For the first time in my parental career I don't have to fret about daytime childcare so I'm enjoying the lie-ins and sneaky late nights as much as Ben is. I don't really know enough about Canadian politics yet to have an informed opinion, although from what I have gleaned there is a lot of organisational 'fat trimming' going on much as the UK played about with some years ago. In which case both sides are probably right. At the moment the teachers are implementing an interesting policy of closing different selections of schools on alternate days of the week. As next week is Ben's safety patrol shift, I'm almost hoping it goes on for a short while. Ten minutes earlier in the morning is hellish when you've been up half the night.

I have sympathy for the working parents though. Opinion at the school gate is pretty anti-teacher, more for the alternate day gambit than the actual strike, which seems to be an annual ritual. Last year the government of

111

Ontario paid organisations like the YMCA to run child-care operations so that parents could get to work. The point of closing different schools on different days this year – those with names beginning with the letter A to M on one day and the rest of the alphabet the next – is to prevent such schemes from being worth setting up, there aren't enough children needing care on any particular day to make it viable to open an ad-hoc centre. This baffles me. If the teachers' argument is with the Province, which it is, I would have thought that costing Mike Harris and his chums money would achieve more than alienating the parents. Maybe I've missed something very obvious and significant, I shall have to keep my ears open at the school gate a little longer.

Anyone who isn't discussing the strike is talking about the weather. Apparently it will snow soon. People are sniffing the air knowledgeably and saying 'snow in the wind' a lot. I have suddenly realised that I ought to buy Ben some winter clothes and that I have no idea how to kit out a child for the kind of arctic conditions that are clearly in the wind. Time for another daft question routine. As usual everyone has different ideas.

'Got to have long underwear!'

'No need for long johns just get snow pants.'

'Don't bother with rubber boots.'

'You'll need rubber boots of course.'

What the hell are snow pants?

We settled for a couple of pairs of thermal long johns to see how they feel, some quilted trousers (I think these are the snow pants) a woolly hat and two pairs of gloves. Why two? We started with a great pair of quilted waterproof ones for snowballing but he can't cycle in them because they slip off the brakes. So now there's another super-duper pair which turn from fingerless gloves into mittens at the touch of a strip of Velcro. Oh and a complicated effort in the boots department involving detachable cuddly fleecy linings. As and when the snows arrive I'll find out just how practical all this lot is. And Ben will find out whether the warming effect of long undies is worth the humour quotient of a hundred music hall gags. And me? Well I have no intention of going out in it although I've seen a rather fetching red fleecy hat that I might indulge in, just to be embarrassing. I had the presence of mind to pack some old thermal vests which date back to my unheated house days. I can press them into service at a pinch. I seem to remember they generate a lot of static electricity so I can spend the winter in a permanent blue haze.

If there's snow in the wind that means it's almost Halloween. Houses are sprouting pumpkins all over their front doorsteps and scary costumes have taken over the shops. I have a big problem with Halloween, mainly because in our part of London it isn't so much a cute kiddies' tradition as an excuse for the local louts to demand money with menaces from elderly ladies. Clearly things are different here. Apparently the cute kiddies' tradition is alive and well and the houses sprouting pumpkins will, by next weekend, be alight with spooky lanterns and full of bags of sweets for scary tots to eat too much of and be sick. I have relented. For the first time ever Ben will be allowed to go trick or treating, scary costume and all. Well, it's part of the transatlantic experience. I'm also going soft in my old age and to prove it he's getting away with bubble gum too.

In continued autumnal mode, we've been sweeping leaves. It all started with the delivery of a leaflet from the City of Kitchener Public Works Department regarding the municipal leaf collection scheme. Why am I surprised? It stands to reason that if you live somewhere with a lot of trees you end up with sufficient leaves to be a municipal issue. It's just one of those tiny but unexpected aspects of living somewhere different that constantly flabbergast me with their obvious necessity. The leaf machine comes round on Monday week. You sweep them into the gutter and a nice man comes and hoovers them up. Can't wait.

* * *

A week later and the Halloween preparations move up a gear. Houses which merely sported pumpkins on their doorsteps are now populated by plastic 'pumpkin people' stuffed with leaves and whimsically arranged reclining in garden chairs on the front porch. I have learned by the way that pumpkins go soft if kept indoors, which is why they live outside. It doesn't explain the faces but no doubt I'll get it in the end. You can even get Halloween garbage bags – pumpkin orange, with manic grins – to fill with leaves in order to liven up your property still further. OK, I admit it, we bought some. I've also been learning the Trick or Treating safety code. It applies to kids and householders alike and it goes along the lines of: 'If a house is all pumpkinned up and has a porch light on, you can stand on the doorstep and ask for sweets, but don't go in. No porch light, don't call, they don't want you.' How sensible. I'm thawing a bit. Might even enjoy it.

Strike's all over by the way. It would now appear that this is a traditional bit of fun to liven up the end of the summer. That's the part I hadn't got, the missing piece of the jigsaw. Everyone's too busy with pumpkins to bother with politics now. Maybe what Britain needs is more national holidays.

* * *

Oh all right then, Halloween was a hoot. Mums and Dads dressed up too, everyone tried to make sure that their garden was scarier than their visitors, Ben has enough sweets to last until Christmas and the schools provided trick or treaters with collecting boxes for UNICEF. I am now an expert in pumpkin carving. There were just a couple of blots on an otherwise jolly occasion, Zuscha has worried herself silly about the poor person sitting in a garden chair on our neighbour's porch:

'She must be very cold.'

'She's made of plastic Zuschy, it's a joke for Halloween, they've stuffed her with leaves, she's not real.'

'Oh OK then. I'm worried about that lady though, she must be very cold.' And on, and on.

I do hope they unstuff her soon. There was also the poor chap who dressed up as a mummy to scare his little visitors, lit a cigarette and set himself on fire. According to *The Record* he won't be OK.

Now that Halloween is over the leaf machines have been. And I have finally sussed the point of the pumpkin bags and plastic people. *The kids fill them with leaves*. Brilliant. They think they are decorating for Halloween but all the time they are really cleaning up ready for the leaf hoover. Having dutifully emptied our leaves from their pumpkin bags into the gutter ready for collection we had been anticipating the machinery with great excitement. It's quite a procedure. First along the route is a lorry with a huge hose on the front, spurting water at the leaf piles. Presumably they fly around less if damped down. Then the hoover lorry lurches by with a huge hose on the back, slurping up little mountain ranges of leaves and churning them into goo. I'm not noted for my enjoyment of outdoor pursuits, I've never quite seen the point of getting sweaty and tired in the garden when you can have a nice sit down in front of the Test Match, but I felt such a glow of civic pride as I contributed to the municipal mulch that I think I may go and sweep some more. Canada sort of does that to you.

And just when you think you've learned it all, you look stupid again. This time it's mobile emergencies. It all started with Theresa asking if I'd put candles in the car yet. The blank look on my face generated a concerned look on hers and she explained in words of one syllable that it was going to snow soon. You can spend a lot of time in your car dying of hypothermia if you break down, get stuck in a snowdrift, encounter a whiteout, etc. etc. A survival kit is the answer.

Feeling irresponsible again, 'OK what do I need?' And the answers are obvious if you give the issue a moment's thought, I just hadn't. The candles are to keep the ambient temperature in the car just above freezing without using the oxygen too fast. It also makes sense to carry waterproof matches, blankets, drinking water, chocolate, a torch, a shovel and some cat litter. Cat litter? I understand it's just the best thing to spread under your wheels for getting out of snowdrifts. The list is made and I have a feeling Theresa will insist on an inspection before she allows us out in the snow.

Theresa has taken our wellbeing to heart in a big way and it is about time I introduced her to you. She arrived in our lives as Theresa-and-Jenny, who visit Zuscha once a week. By way of an experiment. Jenny has learning difficulties and lives in sheltered accommodation, Theresa's job is to take Jenny out and about during the day to give her live-in carer some respite and Jenny some normality and fun. Why do they visit Zuscha once a week? Well Jenny used to love to visit her grandmother. When the old lady died, a huge hole was left in Jenny's life. It seems now that Jenny likes visiting elderly ladies in general, they remind her of her grandma and make her happy. She is possibly the only person who takes a genuine delight in Zuscha's company with no trace of sympathy, condescension or superiority.

Because it began as an experiment, I receive occasional phone calls from Theresa's supervisor to find out how the scheme is working. 'Oh it's such a positive experience' I burble. 'So dignifying for Zuscha to be able to make a contribution to someone else's emotional wellbeing' I witter. I trawl the psychobabble lexicon for superlatives and lo, Theresa-and-Jenny continue to appear in our driveway once a week. I'm not entirely sure that Zuscha gains much from their visits, although Jenny loves us all to bits (and, being serious for a moment, I do think it is a dignifying additional dimension to Zuscha's dwindling experiences) but Theresa is the real reason for my enthusiasm. As soon as she grins her way out of the car – huge red hair following her for another minute or so – my week perks up. Everyone I've met so far is nice but Theresa is fun.

She is one of an indeterminate number of sisters, all resembling Crystal Tipps. We met some of her huge family during The Big One and appear to have been adopted as mascots. Theresa it is who puts me right on candles and chocolate, leaf hoovers and pumpkin bags. It is Theresa to whom I turn with really stupid questions (what are snow pants?) Theresa tells me how patient I sound at putting-the-paper-in-the-toilet time, when I feel anything but. Definitely a positive experience and a successful experiment.

* * *

I realised while shopping for candles and Mars Bars that if it's After Halloween it is therefore Nearly Christmas. Which is strange because in England it's Nearly Christmas if the summer holidays are over. It's a tough assignment sending gifts home when the shops don't start their Christmas displays until the first week in November and the last posting date for surface mail is, yes, the first week in November. I've been spending my time off lurking in shops waiting for one of the boxes due for unpacking to contain Christmas wrapping paper. For days it was everything but. Trees and lights first, followed by large red fabric bows (what for?) then stockings and sacks, kits for trimming your home more tastefully than the neighbours' and finally wrapping paper.

No, come to think of it not finally, the cards have yet to make an appearance, so my packages of presents had to be sent off seasonally wrapped but cardless. I'll know for next year. How many times have I said that? When all the leftover Crimble wrap is selling for next to nothing in January I'll buy lots, then I can spend the first week next November trying to remember where I put it.

As soon as the rush to post prezzies was over I began giving some thought to cards. There are in my life, as I suppose there are in most people's, chums with whom I only correspond at Christmas. Not deliberately you understand, it just happens to be a good time to catch up on the year's news. So three-quarters of my card list don't actually know we're here. That's a lot of writing. The sensible solution would seem to be a long, interesting and jolly epistle from my trusty computer inserted in each card. Unfortunately I have an almost phobic aversion to receiving these round-robin letters from other people and have made my disgust known to all and sundry on a regular basis. The friends to whom I've bitched along the lines of 'who does she think she is? What on earth is so interesting about the kids getting bigger and enjoying cubs that they think I want to read two sides of A4 about it?' will enjoy a good laugh if they finally receive one from me. Trouble is, this time round there's quite a long story to tell, even if I leave out the bit about Ben getting bigger. Maybe I should settle for spreading a bit of Christmas cheer in the form of a hollow chuckle at my expense.

I'm burbling aren't I? Whether or not to compose a duplicated Christmas newsletter isn't really the stuff of which great travelogues are made. It is dawning on me that, as we wait for snow and Christmas and other external punctuations to life, my diary is as desperate for tiny anecdotes as I am for days off. Tiny things define the difference between one day and the next and I feel as though I should be writing snippets for the Reader's Digest.

Life on Planet Alzheimer has blended into a seamless round of sleepless nights and trips to shopping malls for coffee. Some days we look in the pet shop, some days we have extra 'accidents'. It matters a lot to Zuscha whether we see kittens or puppies. It matters a lot to me how big the accidents are. Occasionally she stays in our garden where I can see her long enough for me to put pen to paper. This is a good day. I can prepare her meals and meds in my sleep now…and very often do. Sometimes I stay patient and loving for whole hours at a time, validating each and every moment like the devoted professional I wish I were. Occasionally we fall out, as in an unguarded moment I yell 'NO…!' and immediately regret it during a fraught walk to the bus stop. The things that occupy my mind from day to day aren't worth putting into writing any more, otherwise I'd head each chapter with a put-the-paper-in-the-toilet tally (five, v.good). I'm recounting the diminishing highlights of a shrinking world and just now they are very small indeed.

Today's highlight, a postcard from Scotland. Alison thought I might like to know that she's found a Tobermory there. Maybe the womble wasn't named after the one we went to after all, I never was much good at geography. It explains though why the one we found was full of people in kilts and sporrans playing bagpipes. I thought it was odd at the time but didn't like to ask. Honestly, people as dim as me shouldn't be allowed to globetrot, there ought to be a law or something.

'There's a man besieging the house.'

'Goodness me Zuschy, we'd better check this out, where did you see him?' It's the middle of the day but the curtains are closed. Zuscha is in charge of curtains. She tweaks a corner aside to show me the threat. A man is waiting in a car. His daughter takes guitar lessons from the neighbour opposite.

119

'I see what you mean. I wonder if he might be waiting for someone?'

'Harrumph.'

'I have an idea, shall we look again in a few minutes? He might have gone by then.'

'Sheesh.'

'Sheesh kebab.' She must be very distressed, there is no 'at least'.

'We could have coffee and cookies while we wait.' Another crisis validated. A good day.

ELEVEN

Only Canadians would stand for it

I got lost today. Which makes this a handy moment to have a whinge about Canadian maps. I've always been pretty adept with a map, probably because I like them. I have no patience with the 'left at the lights, right at the pub' brigade, I'm more of a 'give me an address and a map and I'll find it mate' person. But not in Canada. The main highways are pretty self-explanatory, they have numbers and exit signs and stuff. The signage is a bit erratic and takes some getting used to but at least it's the same number from one end to the other and there are signs to be got used to. Off the beaten track is a different story. There are regional roads, county roads and township roads, and each is numbered according to a different system. Sometimes a road has two numbers, because it's a county road and a regional road at one and the same time. Which is fine if the number on the road sign happens to match the one your map, which it generally doesn't, or if the turning you want has a sign at all, which it generally won't. Different funding you see. The local authority pays for the road signs, so they will label a road with its local number. Maps aren't paid for by municipalities, so they opt to use the regional numbering system. It makes perfect sense until you want to try and go anywhere.

Of course some districts tend to eschew the road sign completely, presumably this represents a significant municipal saving. It is a natural British assumption that an unlabelled track isn't really a road and won't go anywhere you'd want to get to, so there's bound to be a signposted one further on. I'm getting quite adept at the sort of ill-tempered U-turn required when it turns out that the almost-junction a mile or so back probably was the turning you wanted after all. Ben is learning to swear.

And then there's the road name issue. People only ever use half a road name here, so there's obviously no point in cartographers being picky. The place you want is on King and Weber, or Lancaster and Victoria. No-one cares whether you mean Road, Avenue, Street or Drive. Being used to London – where for every Regent or Cavendish there's a Road, an Avenue, a Crescent, a Street and very probably a Square and a Mews – I tend to assume that maps will get the road names right even if they sport conflicting numbers.

So when, and this is the point in case you were wondering, this morning I passed a country lane marked Reichtel Drive, I naively assumed that the Reichtel Road I was looking for would be a little further on. Abrupt U-turn when it became apparent that the difference between a road and a drive is an insignificant detail to the masters of uncertainty at Allmaps Canada Ltd. I recently read Bill Bryson waxing lyrical about the joys of Ordnance Survey maps. Now I understand. Ben knows not to repeat at school anything he hears while Mummy is driving.

We were trying to find a craft fair. I'm taking a bit of an interest in the sudden appearance of craft fair listings in the local papers, it looks as though there is money to be made in the run up to Christmas if you're at all handy in the 'making something from bits of nothing' department. I used to dabble a bit so was dead keen to find out what sells and how much for, with a view to making a killing next year.

The fair, once we found it, was an eye opener. A roughly equal mix of stunning craftsmanship and total junk. Selling with equal speed. I place my own efforts in neither category I should point out but am now inspired to fill the empty hours more profitably. Oddly enough, the stalls selling out fastest were the ones full of things that anyone could make for themselves if so minded. The baskets of pinecones sprayed gold and interspersed with little lights sold out in a couple of hours. Far more popular than the intricate work of talented wood turners and lace makers, each project blossoming from a lifetime's devotion to beauty and a passion for keeping such precious skills alive. I don't understand this but am suddenly minded to settle here for ever and learn to make lace and turn wood. I can leave the blacksmithing to Ben.

I should add by the way that the red bows (what for?) that I spotted in the shops last week are now beginning to appear on people's gateposts. Yes, we're not half way through November and the Christmas decorations are out. It's as though houses must be 'trimmed' for something the year round. As soon as one festival ends, the decorations for the next appear post haste. On the gatepost. Gatepost haste? During the summer it was cutesy little windmills and wooden shepherdesses hiding coyly in the herbaceous borders, there were decorative corncobs for Thanksgiving and I think I may have mentioned the pumpkins. Gosh, I wonder if there'll be Easter bunnies. Ben is a convert and doesn't want ours to be the only house in the street without Stuff for Christmas. I am playing for time.

* * *

No snow yet but we've found some ice. There's free rink outside Kitchener City hall where the fountains used to be, the council ice over their ornamental pond every winter as a public amenity. Isn't that nice? It's well maintained and marshalled, floodlit after dark, there's music and toilets, changing room and a Zamboni, complete with grumpy driver. Ben and I dashed out to equip ourselves with second hand ice skates. Every sports shop has a cheapo second-hand skate exchange in the basement because all the kids need new ones each year. I wouldn't dream of such extravagance at home but with free skating down the road all winter it just had to be done.

I have just about forgiven him for showing me up on our first visit. Hardly had the words 'hang on to me Ben, you've never skated before and I used to be quite good so I'll show you how' left my lips when I was unaccountably sitting down and he was off as though born with skates on his feet.

It's a great place to see everybody and his nephew out and about. Tiny tots are shuffling about hanging onto little plastic hockey goals which double as ice-rink walking frames. They then graduate to brilliant little double bladed skates which strap onto their toddler shoes. I wonder if they come in size seven. Older kids are practising figures, adults are gently blowing away the cobwebs and budding hockey players weave carefully in and out of us all. The nicest time to be there is just before dusk. Then, as the air gets that smoky edge, just before it gets even colder, you can watch the Christmas lights flicker on tree by tree along the High Street. Magical.

Speaking of Christmas lights, the houses that had red bows on their gateposts last week now have coloured lights all over the roof as well. And little wooden sleighs by the chimney. And plastic snowmen on the lawns. Now correct me if I'm wrong but this is Canada. It will snow. Surely your actual snow snowman will be free? I am becoming more and more bemused by the exploits of all these serial house-trimmers. The words 'vulgar' and 'kitsch' came to mind so often this week that I am beginning to dislike my attitude even more than I dislike the lights. I had a ponder along the lines of 'why don't we do this at home then?' and concluded that most of the stuff would be disappear overnight if we did. Feeling less superior as a result.

Zuscha is fascinated by the lights on our neighbour's roof. She spends her evenings gazing out of the window, calling me to admire them with her several times an hour. Unusually, she remembers them from day to day. And spending her nocturnal prowling time wondering where they've gone. Very loudly.

The Record has Christmas on its mind just now. Spare a thought for the 200 workers laid off at this time of year from the Colonial Cookies plant. So many people go on diets after the festive season that an annual cookie-making slowdown means layoffs all-round. I have trouble comprehending the number of people required to diet for this to be necessary. Especially since Canadians seem to turn out a bit bigger than the average Brit. The same edition (World News section, natch) gleefully reported problems finding fat enough Santa Clauses (Clausi?) in England. Too many actors are eating salad, which means that Santa-sized candidates are hard to find and 'kids can spot padding'. Maybe budding British Santas should be sent to Canada to eat biscuits as part of a mutual employment protection scheme. I feel a letter coming on.

The bank is all prettied up for the festivities too. I took Zuscha with me on one of our afternoon expeditions. I sat her down in a comfy chair in the waiting area before joining the queue. My trouble-antennae must have had the day off because I completely failed to notice the rather attractive silk Poinsettia arrangement in a tub next to her chair. It took her about as long to rip all the red bits off as it took me to get served. She ambled up to the counter to join me and – with a proudly happy smile – tipped glorious and abundant handfuls of red silk leaves all over our bank book. The cornucopia spilled generously into the bank teller's lap. 'I'm awfully sorry' didn't seem adequate somehow, so I made the mistake of embarrassed people everywhere and began to wibble. When I found myself explaining to the entire bank – with demonstrations – how easy it would be to stick the red bits back onto the stalks above the green bits again I realised I had probably said enough.

That evening Ben's simmering ear infection went into orbit. One of those screaming in pain efforts that comes on suddenly just after you've decided to see a doctor tomorrow if it doesn't improve and sent the Zuscha-sitter away. In the end I had to bundle all of us into the car and transport the entire household to the local walk-in clinic. Ontario doesn't have family doctors. Well, that's not strictly true, they exist but they're an endangered species. If you settled here during the early fifties you may have a family doctor by now. The rest of us make do with walk-in clinics.

I had my doubts about the medical expertise we were likely to encounter at one of these, equating the sort of doctors who might work in one with late-night locums at home but I couldn't have been more wrong. The clinics tend to take their doctors fresh from medical school. They are therefore enthusiastic, up-to-date and trained to talk to people. The young man who saw Ben (after we'd installed Zuscha contentedly in the waiting room with a magazine with pictures of kittens and reassured the receptionist that I would leap into action should she show any sign of absconding) was magnificent. He spent ages discussing with me which would be the most effective antibiotic bearing in mind all out family allergies, the need to bash what he described as a spectacular infection really hard and Ben's diminutive size for his age. He then found a free sample to get us through the night so that we wouldn't have to drag Zuscha to the pharmacy and do all the magazine-with-kittens stuff over again. Impressed is inadequate really.

Unimpressed is pretty inadequate too, for my response to the cost of said antibiotics when we did get to a drugstore the following day. The five-pounds-something you pay at home for each item is about what the chemist charges here to look at your prescription. A sort of pharmaceutical call-out charge. Then you pay for the medication as well. One bottle of pink stuff came to forty-three dollars. That's about twenty quid. I shall stop moaning about the NHS forthwith.

We have next weekend off to go and see the Christmas lights at Niagara Falls. At least I won't be tempted into the purchase of tacky souvenirs, most of my available cash has disappeared on medicine.

(The lights will have to be pretty special to beat Kitchener's Victoria Park. We drifted along one evening to see what everyone was raving about and were instantly transported to fairyland. It's a pretty park anyway, with a lake under the trees and nice little wooden bridges dotted about. With lights strung in the trees and across the bridges all reflecting in the water the effect was stunning. We both giggled out loud, just because it was so pretty. And I'm not generally a giggling out loud because things are pretty sort of person.)

While moaning about money I may as well go the whole hog and confess that a cheque bounced this week. It bounced because I ordered a chequebook. My account balance wasn't huge, or even healthy but it did just about cover the cheque I'd written for Ben's chess lessons while awaiting my wages, which have been arriving a little erratically of late. Once the bank had charged me for the privilege of owning one of their chequebooks however, sneakily deducting the princely sum of twelve dollars from my account, the cheque bounced. They then charged me for returning the cheque, thus placing me in the red and are now charging me for the resultant overdraft. And for writing and telling me about it. Coming from a land where banks decided a long time ago that the privilege of having your money to play with was something for which they should pay you, I am not amused. There's no point in complaining of course, it'll be in the small print somewhere. And I thought transaction charges were scandalous. Only Canadians would stand for it.

They don't seem to get up in arms about anything, these supremely polite people – bank charges, useless maps, exporting all the best cheese – they just ask you how you are and carry on having nice lives. Maybe it has something to do with having Father Christmas as a citizen, could he be a role model too? Did you know Father Christmas was a Canadian? The North Pole is geographically in Canada, ergo Santa is a local. We're terribly pleased and rather relieved as it helps with the chimney situation. We don't have one at our current abode and Ben was beginning to fret about what to send his letter up. Then the TV adverts started publicising Santa's address, we will not require air-mail this year. There is even a postcode, which is naturally enough H0H 0H0. All letters will receive a reply from the great man himself and we are eagerly awaiting ours. The replies are written by public-spirited post office volunteers, not remarkable in itself – I seem to recall there are such kindly people at home too – what impresses me particularly is that the TV adverts for this little scheme are sponsored by a charitable literacy campaign. It gets kids writing letters. I do think that's rather neat.

No I don't. I don't think anything is neat unless it's tidy. The literacy campaign may be clever, kind, impressive, splendid or possibly fab but I can't justify picking up neat as an expression of approval. I don't wish to appear supercilious about English English, I'm gradually converting to Canada-speak in order to be understood in the shops but neat is a concession too far. I shall have to get a moneybox and slip in a quarter every time I lapse. It'll help with all the bank charges.

Ben and I have decided to try and festive-up the house a bit. We dug around in the basement and found a moth-eaten old wreath and a small, scruffy Christmas tree. We did our best and the house began to look positively jolly for a while.

The festive wreckage began with the wreath. Zuscha has embarked on a nocturnal mission to destroy it in stages. I repair it each morning and hang it back on the front door so that ours won't be the only house without Stuff. (I put my foot down with regard to fairy lights by the way, not so much an aesthetic decision as a ladder-climbing one in the end.) Each day there is a little less wreath to repair. 'Oh well' we thought, 'at least the Christmas tree looks safe enough.' And it was. Until last night. Ben is upset. With all signs of the festive season demolished beyond repair we have given up, apart from the tiny raffia reindeer secreted in Ben's room. I've promised him that the very next Christmas we spend in a place of our own we'll have the biggest real tree we can fit through the door. And we will, because I'm upset too.

That reindeer can get up to some high jinks though, a new naughtiness every night. Sometimes he snaffles a tiny glass of wine, sometimes he is to be found sitting in an empty box of Smarties, occasionally he clambers into bed with Ben just to be awkward. He is too tiny to feature in Zuscha's world as she cruises around at night and is therefore safe from interference. He is almost as much fun as a tree and I have a feeling I will be dreaming up new nocturnal high jinks for him every Christmas until Ben is thirty-five.

Systematic demolition seems to be Zuscha's main preoccupation just now. She sees each project doggedly through to its completion, regardless of how long it takes.

Some, like the mission to remove every button from a favourite shirt, can be completed in an evening. Others take a little longer. The removal of an interesting wire in our mailbox kept her occupied for days. I have been wondering what purpose it used to serve as nothing seems to have stopped working yet, no doubt I will find out sooner or later. I thought I'd hit the jackpot with the shirt buttons. The task generated such a lovely quiet evening that I sewed them all back on again to keep her amused the following night but Zuscha is not so easily manipulated. Anything I deliberately set up for demolition is instantly no longer worthy of her attention. I ought to know better by now, life on Planet Alzheimer isn't allowed to be in any way predictable.

We are anxiously awaiting snow. Victoria Park will be even prettier once the lake freezes but this shows no sign of occurring. Which is not as it should be. Each night on the News we hear that the weather has broken new records. The clothing stores are in desperate straits, winter coats and boots aren't selling at all well but we're not sorry because Niagara in an unseasonably warm December was utterly glorious. Cold enough to blow the cobwebs away and sunny enough to generate those legendary rainbows.

When I first saw postcards and souvenirs of the Falls, I assumed the rainbows had been touched in. When my photos came back from the developers after our first visit I realised they hadn't. As the sun shines on the mist that rises from the pressure of water on the river below, little rainbows appear all over the place. Legend has it that the Maid of the Mist – a native girl who took her kayak over the Falls rather than be married (and who can blame her?) lives on in the rainbows and grants good fortune to those who see her. Having accidentally photographed some last time, rainbow snapping was high on the agenda for this visit. And the Maid kindly provided us with the most perfect specimen I have ever, ever seen. Truly. A perfect bow, beginning in the

Falls, arching majestically across the heavens and ending in the car park. We both threw in a dime and made a wish. Soppy or what?

Also high on the agenda this weekend was a furtherance of Ben's quest for the finest meatball in the land. It started with his first dish of spaghetti and meatballs, not a common combination at home but pretty standard fare over here. I sang him the song naturally. Now he always orders spaghetti and meatballs if he can and we both sing the song.

He has begun a rating system with marks out of ten for meatball scrumptiousness. The pizzeria we found on Saturday night only scored five. Not a patch on our local Sunday Brunch haunt (eight out of ten). The meal was nonetheless memorable because after our ritual rendition of the song – quietly of course – Ben actually sneezed. The pair of us dissolved into the sort of helpless giggling usually reserved for the junior playground. Generally when we eat out we make friends with everyone in the place on the basis that Ben has a cute accent. This time we made friends all round because he has such a dirty laugh. *Plus ça change.*

We saw the Christmas lights. Very spectacular they are too, or would have been anywhere else. I did find myself wondering why anyone would want to try to create something spectacular by, near or around a place so effortlessly spectacular in its own right. But then they do it to attract the tourists. We're tourists and we went to see them. So it works.

The eruption of twinkly lights is not the only harbinger of impending festivities. Ben's school concert has been and gone and I now know that it is not Nearly Christmas, it is Nearly Winter Holiday. I have displayed my ignorance again and ought to report another huge culture shock. Schools in Harringay are allowed to have Christmas, complete with nativity plays and carols, as long as they pay equal attention to other religious festivals. Ben has a reasonable working knowledge of Divali, Eid and Yom Kippur as a result. This suits me fairly well, a nose round the world's major religions seems a good method of enabling kids to choose their own belief system (or absence thereof) in the fullness of time.

Here the purpose of the festive season is left sufficiently vague to cover all possible ways of celebrating the middle of winter. 'Happy Holidays' is the cry, in shops, on TV and in greetings cards. The school show was careful not to nod in the direction of one religion more than any others and therefore majored on Santa getting stuck down various chimneys and being rescued by a bunch of helpful chimney-sweeps. Ben was in the choir and he – and I – enjoyed it thoroughly but I felt somehow let down by the absence of baby Jesus and raffia donkeys.

I can see the multicultural point but it does seem to take kids further away than ever from the idea that, whatever your religion, 'holidays' are about more than presents and food. Thinking back to the Harringay approach, some parents objected violently to their children being taught about other faiths, so I suppose neither method is foolproof. I just like to cry when the angel's wings fall off and Mary picks her nose.

Sad news in *The Record* this week. And a lot of buck passing. It is as yet unclear whether Federal Express or US Customs were responsible for putting 10,000 year old glacier samples in the fridge rather than the freezer in transit over the border. Yes, a puddle of water arrived at Penn. State University and the boffins are not happy. I know it's not funny really.

TWELVE

Odd, the rituals you miss

Snow. Just in time for Christmas. At last Ben can stop tobogganing round the house and get to drop wet clothes all over the place instead. I understand the thing with the fairy lights now. The street may have looked silly before it snowed but now it's utterly delightful. It helps with navigation too, breaking up the white expanses so that you can see where the streets are. Some side roads even colour co-ordinate their houses so that alternate houses match. It is neither naff nor kitsch, it's brilliant. When all the road signs are snowed over, you can head for the one past the blue and white road. I wish now – but then I'll know for next year.

The snow has produced a new addition to my repertoire of Canadian experiences, shovelling the sidewalk. There's a by-law to make sure you do. Just now it's still enough of a novelty to be enjoyable, the stuff isn't too deep yet and it's rather good exercise, although I can imagine getting pretty sick of the job sooner or later, especially if we cop a malicious snow-plough driver. According to the neighbours these legendary chaps hide round the corner until you've finished shovelling your driveway nice and clean, then they gleefully deposit tons of packed snow from the road all over your handiwork. Can't wait.

The wonderful white stuff adds a new dimension to Christmas shopping too. Struggling with bags and boxes is much more fun when added to the fight with scarves and gloves and extraneous fleecy apparatus. Now that it's cold you see, it's really cold. The wind chill generated a cool (and I use the word advisedly) minus 21 degrees yesterday, so it's hat, scarf and gloves for the short dash from car park to shopping mall, followed by half an hour disrobing inside because the shops are warm, leaving no hands free for jolly goodies of the giftly sort.

Last-minute Christmas shopping would appear to be the same the world over though which is faintly reassuring. I notice that the famous Canadian politeness takes a bit of a bashing when the shops are due to close and everyone needs the same parking space in order to buy something nasty for Great Aunt Nancy.

Here's something that isn't the same. Adverts on TV for children's toys. British advertisers have to confess their prices up front don't they? I only twigged this when buying a radio-controlled car that Ben had requested from Santa. I've watched the ad with him several times, I'm sure I'd have noticed the price had they mentioned it, it's huge. No choice now. And what's more it needs a battery charger. I am developing a touch of the bah-humbugs. Oddly enough, in most other areas advertisers have to confess to a lot here that they get away with at home. Side effects for example. Medication commercials have to list every possible known reaction in order to be legal, leading to some whimsical ads with ludicrously disproportionate amounts of air time devoted to what can go wrong, something along the lines of:

Snoozy-woozy, your wonderful bed-time friend, wave goodbye to sleepless nights! If you are taking any other medications or have any allergies, consult your doctor before taking this medication. Known side-effects can include dizziness, nausea, stomach cramps, weight gain, hives, impotence, temporary blindness and Lassa Fever.

OK, I made up the last few but how on earth they get away with keeping the price of kiddies' toys a secret is beyond me.

Ben asked me what I wanted for Christmas. I've told him I'd like a pepper mill. I really do want one too. Clearly Zuscha wasn't a freshly ground pepper sort of person because there isn't one here and I miss mine terribly. I like black pepper on my fried eggs you see. This dates back to a series of deep and meaningful conversations with my first ever ambulance crewmate on quiet night shifts way back in another lifetime. One is often peckish on a night shift, the conversations regularly turn to food. In this case, the ultimate fried egg. We agreed that the only way to create the truly great fried egg experience is to grind your pepper freshly over it while it cooks and that sprinkling some ready ground on afterwards (whether white or black) diminishes the dish in criminal manner. A properly fried and peppered egg takes me right back to younger, fitter and more heroic days and makes me happy, so I currently get a little wave of homesickness every time I fry an egg. Odd, the rituals you miss. Please bear in mind as you assess my level of sanity that whole weeks go by during which a nicely fried egg is the most interesting thing that happens during the day. I know I could buy a pepper mill but I've never needed to before – I had three as wedding presents – so I never think of it. I do hope Santa helps Ben find a nice one, it might make up for the total absence of mince pies.

Why don't Canadians have mince pies? I assumed they were part of the NATO Standard Christmas. I'd make my own if I could find any jars of mince in the shops but no-one knows what I am talking about and I have regretfully come to the conclusion that this will be a mince-pie-free Yule. Odd, the rituals you miss.

By way of a break from mince pie hunting we've been sampling more Christmas lights, Victoria Park (of the fairyland appearance) is Kitchener's pride and joy. Waterloo Park, not unreasonably, is Waterloo's fave pretty place. Generally we prefer it, it has a little petting zoo, peacocks and a splash park and Waterloo's oldest building – a wooden school house, they're very proud of it and move it about from time to time, the better to make sure everyone gets to admire it. But in the Christmas light department we have voted it a little substandard, a tad modern for out taste, neon Santas and multicoloured dinosaurs and the like. Seeing them in style however made for a grand treat all the same. Wandering about in a biting wind that finds all the gaps in your fleecy things, we happened upon a notice that said Trolley Stop. The trolley in question turned out to be horse-drawn, heated, brilliant fun and free. We clippety-clopped round the Christmas lights singing carols led with gusto by our trolley driver and feeling positively festive. Despite our mince-pielessness.

We went to a party on Christmas Eve. As Theresa's family's adopted mascots we were invited to join them at their traditional bash hosted by another Crystal Tipps called Susan, who welcomed us with warmth and hugs. Because her sister likes us. The occasion involved all the adults periodically falling silent as the children listen in to radio bulletins on Santa's progress. I had to have it carefully explained but I now understand how they do it. NORAD satellites track the sleigh using radiation from Rudolph's nose and all local radio stations carry regular updates. It is, I'm told, the traditional way to terrify children into bed. We left for home when the great man was somewhere near Halifax.

We turned up our noses however at the other great Canadian Christmas tradition of leaving out milk and cookies for Santa. At home he gets sherry and mince pies. Since this establishment doesn't have sherry-drinking visitors – and let's face it, we all only buy sherry to give to visitors – and, well, I think I may have mentioned the mince pie famine, we treated him to a small glass of Cinnamon Schnapps and a large slice of buttered Pannetone. The Cinnamon Schnapps had been an early festive gift from Alison, presented to me before we left England to hide away for toasting absent friends on Christmas Day. Had I known then how much it would haunt future endeavours I'd have given Santa a much larger glassful. Or possibly the whole bottle, but I digress.

We also left out the usual nine carrots. Pat, who is home for the holidays – hers this time, not mine – looked a little bemused as I carefully nibbled round carrot tops in the early hours of Christmas morning to make it look as though the reindeer had eaten them. Doesn't everyone do this? Actually we were a little restrained this year. Usually Ben persuades me to leave out a cracker for Santa as well and a card for Rudolph if it's not foggy. I honestly don't know who's conning who. Have you ever tried to pull a cracker Very Quietly after too much of Santa's sherry? Take it from me, it's not easy.

Remember the battery charger? I'd felt so clever, reading the packaging in advance and noticing that we needed one so that Ben could play with his car on Christmas morning. Pity I didn't read the instructions after I bought it, especially the bit about charging for five hours. Fortunately Santa had thought of several other goodies to keep hyper people quiet

Carolyn Steele

until tobogganing time. There was food to eat of course and more prezzies and telling Zuscha we thought it might be Christmas sometime soon so we might as well unwrap some things. (Well, not knowing what day it is pretty demeaning, so Pat and I just never know what day it is either.) The five hours passed tolerably fast. With huge excitement we placed our freshly charged battery in the radio control unit. Nothing happened.

Clearly one of the elves had misread the box. The other battery was the one that needed a charger. The one that went in the car. The one we didn't have. If I ever find that elf I'm going to give him a serious talking to.

Ben gave me a necklace. He'd chosen the beads. It's very pretty. Not a peppermill but maybe he decided that a kitchen gadget wasn't exciting enough for a prezzie. Unusual for a chap, I do hope he doesn't change when he's married.

The day passed tolerably well in the end, it felt a bit odd at first as Christmases somewhere new always do but as soon as Theresa and co. collected us for our first tobogganing lessons it was so totally out of the ordinary that we began to have fun again.

Boxing Day dawned bright and sunny so we went skating to complete the winter sports collection. Now that we have skated and tobogganed we know we've had a proper white Christmas. Then all the shops opened up again, jam-packed with bargain hunters, so it's back to the way things are at home. Particularly since a fellow skater reminded me that Kitchener boasts a branch of *Marks and Spencer*. I'd forgotten. I don't usually go there, I'm generally more interested in learning to shop Canadian than recreating home but Christmas is different, so I popped along as soon as they opened and sure enough the mince pies were half price. I bought a pack for everyone who'd put up with me bemoaning their absence. Nobody liked them much.

* * *

My winter education is progressing nicely. The local radio station has begun to broadcast esoteric weather warnings that everyone understands except me. I now know that 'flash freeze between six and seven' means that the sloppy slush on the roads when we pop into *Gatto's* for a veggie burger and fries (onion rings, the sauerkraut-to-die-for and special sauce on the side) will be a sheet of ice by the time we emerge to drive home. If I've got this right, a flash freeze happens when the sky clears suddenly and the temperature drops too fast for slush to dry out. Zero to minus twelve in less than an hour does the trick very nicely. Yup it's getting cold.

* * *

New Year's Eve was different. We sampled Kitchener's City Hall's Festival of the Night: 'a non-alcoholic, family New Year's Eve celebration'. Until this year I knew of three basic ways to see in the new year; earning double time picking up drunk and injured revellers, paying double time to a baby-sitter in order to go out and get drunk and preferably not injured oneself or sitting at home alone with a bottle of gin and Clive James on the telly. The idea of a municipally-sponsored, city-centre family party is an old one here and it works.

Free skating, live music, dancing, hot drinks and pizzas outside, face painting and kiddies' entertainers indoors, lots to see and do. Ben loved the ice sculptures and I was rather taken with the huge banner on the wall on which the populace are encouraged to scribble their New Year's resolutions. I was even more taken with the whimsical idea of posting last year's resolution banner on the opposite wall so that you could look up your failures and cringe.

It was a bit cold for a party to be honest. Being mainly outside. We took all the advice we could collate on the subject of keeping warm but missed out on one vital element, super-cold drinks. Carefully layered with ears covered and draughty gaps plugged, Ben got a bit too thirsty after his pizza for hot chocolate so I found him a Coke. Too late, Theresa in her fount-of-all-wisdom-cold-weather-wise guise said 'Oh don't drink that too fast, it's colder that usual and you'll make yourself sick. See the ice crystals forming in the bottle?'

We came home early a bit queasy. Which was fine, it enabled me to have a beer in my hand as midnight struck. For once I allowed myself a self indulgent ponder. (Since the Big One I have tried to resist the temptation to think too hard about anything.) Last New Year's Eve my brand new diary was empty. It was a metaphor for my future, life was going nowhere. I don't quite know what Planet Alzheimer is a metaphor for but we appear to be in a continual state of going somewhere these days. Grabbing life by the scruff of the neck is an odd thing to do in your 40s but I suppose it beats slippers and Coronation Street. Most of the time. I'm almost more excited than scared but not quite.

* * *

By the way, we've had a tad more snow. And I'm learning. No sooner had I twigged the difference between a flurry and a squall, I had the opportunity to suss the difference between a squall and a blizzard. Eleven inches overnight is a blizzard, which means I must learn to shovel properly. It would appear that we've only been playing at it so far. It felt real enough at the time but what do I know? The protocol seems a little bizarre to a newcomer but I understand it's a steep learning curve.

First you shovel your way out of the drive, carefully not walking on any of it first because that packs it down and makes it heavier. To this end the purists try to beat the mailman to it, otherwise he treads on it for you. Then you wait for the snowplough driver to appear. He shovels all the snow from the road into a little mountain range that plugs the space you've just shovelled in your driveway. Then you shovel the snowplough's shovellings before they freeze into an ice sleeping policeman where the drive meets the road. Otherwise the car won't go anywhere before April. Then, when you're exhausted, you do the sidewalk. Because there's a bye-law.

Waiting for the snowplough to pass by before you start is so that you only have to shovel once is, counter-intuitively, a Bad Thing. The road shovellings are heavy with grit and salt and stuff. It's easier back-muscle-wise to clear the bottom layer while it's all nice and powdery. Not that my back is particularly cognisant of the difference just now.

Burying the fire hydrant in snow is also a Bad Thing. Firemen don't like having to dig it out during an emergency. Responsible citizen that I am, I carefully kept my driveside heap of shovellings about an inch below the hydrant's workings. I still have a UK mind, I am expecting it to melt soon. It's snowed again now of course. The snow piles up for months here. The mountain has grown. More shovelling.

I have also leaned that British Rail were right, there are different types of snow. This stuff is no good for snowmen. We tried. According to Theresa, who is herself learning that we need to have things explained carefully that she inhaled as a child, snowman snow happens at zero or thereabouts when the snow is wet enough to stick together. At minus a lot the stuff is too dry. And what's more, 'you know it's really cold when the snow squeaks under your feet and your nose hairs freeze.' Oddly enough I can tell if it's really cold without the sound effects. Clearly I am becoming an expert.

* * *

Goodness me, it's still snowing. According to the statisticians we had more snow last week than in the whole of the previous winter. According to the neighbours 'well you did want to experience a real Canadian winter didn't you?'

El Nino is to blame. Or possibly me. Each day there's more. And more. And then a little sprinkle more.

I'm seeing more of the neighbours now than ever, we're all out shovelling at about the same time, pre or post plough, and much neighbourliness accompanies the shovelling routine. Families with teenaged kids loan them out to the people who need to get to work, with pocket money changing hands naturally. The rest of us club together to dig out the old folks. A wonderful man from along the road and round the corner somewhere has appeared with a little pavement sized sit-upon snowplough. He clears one sidewalk for everyone on the way to his Mum's and the other on the way back. He is universally adored.

The local radio station has a 'snow-desk' report twice an hour. It covers road conditions, school and business closures, flight delays etc. We have to tune in at seven-fifteen in the morning to check if Ben's school is open. On the morning after the first 'big dump' the snow-desk bulletin ran along the lines of, 'these roads are closed, these schools are closed and this is how many people died shovelling yesterday.' The newspapers are running columns on safe shovelling along with a checklist of heart attack symptoms. It really is that bad. Toronto and Buffalo, just over the border, have called in the military after grinding to a halt. K/W kept moving fairly well during the initial crisis, mainly because people tend not to park out on the roads here like they have to in the bigger cities. We've all got posh driveways. They're hard work to shovel but at least the snowploughs can get by to clear the streets. Now the sheer volume of white stuff they're shifting is causing problems because there's nowhere left to put it all. The snow dump is full and the hunt is on for a municipal overflow. I love the idea of a snow dump. We have to go and see it. No-one understands this.

I'm running out of places to put it all too. Once a heap of snow is up to your shoulders, each shovelful has to go over your head to add to it, which makes even a light fall hard work to clear. And no-one can see you pulling your car out of the drive from behind it either. The biggest danger on the road isn't slippery bits, it's cars suddenly appearing from behind enormous piles of snow. So I've started housekeeping the heaps. I'm lopping the tops off, spreading them out, neatening the corners, rounding the edges, like a cross between bakery and sculpture. Next week the Henry Moore, or possibly a peacock.

The Record reports the year's first incident of snow rage. Yes, someone has finally smacked a snowplough driver. We all know they're only doing their job but I have to admit to wondering how they know I have to get Zuscha somewhere in the car in five minutes' time. I have a new ambition now. I want to drive a snowplough, I couldn't be any worse at it than I am at tobogganing. Ben lent me his new super-duper version (with brakes) at the weekend. Another steep learning curve, this one with a snowdrift at the bottom. I spent more time than is consistent with middle-aged motherly dignity upside down in it, giggling too helplessly to move and wondering how I'd managed to collect quite so much snow up my nose and sleeves. Apparently my problem has to do with weight distribution. It was ever thus.

It's getting colder too. The snow-desk suggested today that if your child's school was open (Ben's won't give in) you might want to get the car out. At minus twenty-three – with a wind chill making it feel like minus thirty-five – exposed skin freezes in less than two minutes, they said. I took Ben to school in the car.

Big news. There's a school talent show next month. Cue for another knock-em-dead magic show. The script is written, the rehearsals under way and a sneaky new trick involving a vase of water and an unwary teacher is under construction. The event will be directed by the French teacher. *Madame* is to vet the scripts next week. Hope the new trick gets through.

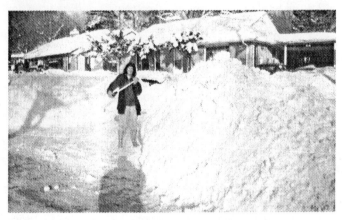

Learning to shovel

THIRTEEN

Maple syrup tinted specs

I've applied to be a Block Parent. I've been a little bemused by signs all over the place saying 'This is a Block Parent neighbourhood' for a while now and decided it was time to make enquiries. Block parents, I can now report, are people who've been checked out by the police as law abiding, safe and sensible. They then display a sign in the window when they're at home. The sign means that any child in trouble will be safe calling at your home for help. What a great idea. Why don't we do it? Hope I pass the checks. I doubt somehow that the K/W police will turn up anything the Immigration authorities couldn't, so with any luck I'm on my way to block parenthood and a spot of Canadian good citizenship to add to my assiduous shovelling.

Actually there have been several changes to the snow situation this week. The first thing to happen was that whole days went by without any fresh snowfall. This gave the ploughs time to pootle about housekeeping their heaps and managing the municipal snow-topiary, much as I've been rearranging mine. Mountain ranges by the roadside turned into sheer cliff faces as the ploughs neatened their edges and mitred their corners, taking the shavings to the newly opened overflow snow dump. They decided to tidy our road overnight. So even on days when no snow fell there were still snowplough droppings to attend to, solid ice by the morning. The street rang to the merry sound of people hammering their ice sleeping policemen to bits with picks and shovels before driving to work.

Then it warmed up a little. Then it began to rain. Some of the snow from the tops of the heaps thawed and joined the rain in the street. The bottoms of the heaps remained in tact because, being so big, they are very cold in the middle. Aren't I the expert? The point of this scientific discourse is that flooding ensues if you don't dig out the drains. Toronto has its soldiers doing just that.

Thawing snow is more dangerous than you'd suppose. It generates the most fantastic icicles, I've been busy photographing them, it didn't occur to me until I read it in the papers that the arty phenomenon I'm happily snapping is pretty lethal when falling from a skyscraper. There are enormous ice stilettos dropping from buildings all over Toronto. Then one has the sheet ice which covers the roads when floodwater freezes overnight to contend with. And the potholes. A huge one opened up suddenly on the outside lane of our main highway this week, due to the road freezing and thawing too fast. That one caused a road closure, smaller ones just terrify unwary cyclists. I'm still fascinated by the Ontario winter. Does it show?

Parts of Canada more used to this kind of snowfall than us lily-livered southerners have had a good laugh at the crises. The TV news delights in quoting residents of Montreal, who think the fuss in Toronto is just too funny for words. 'This is Canada' they chortle 'it snows'. Torontonians delighted in a quiet return chortle when the roof of Montreal's much prized new Olympic stadium collapsed. Too much snow apparently.

Zuscha isn't chortling. She fumes and swears at the white stuff. She knows it's stopping her gardening but isn't quite on top of the details. She spends long hours at the window shaking her fists at the icicles. While the ground was white she wouldn't venture out but as soon as the thaw set in she was off to pursue her favourite winter pastime of sweeping rainwater away down the street. I haven't got to the bottom of this little obsession yet but there's no stopping her.

Generally it's safe enough so long as I dress her in a day-glow raincoat and head her off before the bottom of our road. It's a cul-de-sac and everyone who lives on the street drives slowly – anticipating the little day-glow rainsweeping lady – but just now she's not safe anywhere. Five-foot high snow banks along the roadside ensure she can't be seen by the most careful of drivers whatever she's wearing. Icy patches mean that drivers who do see her are as likely to mow her down as not.

Explanations, pleadings and arguments have got me nowhere. Sweeping rainwater is what she does. This may sound unkind but I've taken to making sure she goes out a little underdressed, so that a couple of minutes later I can join her sweeping, bring up the subject of feeling cold and we can come indoors again. It seems kinder than the alternative.

* * *

Plans for the talent show continue apace. We were a little concerned that *Madame* might axe the water gag but *Madame* appears to have a sense of humour. She has not only passed the script as submitted but promised to keep the secret. We are both terribly excited.

Another week, another weird weather phenomenon. This week it's freezing rain. The radio warning sounded serious and all the schools immediately cancelled all their buses. I wondered why people accustomed to foul weather were in such a flat spin.

'What's freezing rain?' Ben asked. I did my finest impression of an all-knowing parent, 'Dunno, bit like hail I suppose.'

It's not anything like hail. Hail is hail. Freezing rain is, well, stunningly beautiful and terrifyingly dangerous. I'll engage scientific mode for a sentence or two and then go and lay down in a darkened room.

The temperature at ground level has to be just about zero with a warm front passing high overhead. What starts as rain when it leaves its cloudy home freezes as it lands. Not quite snow, or slush or ice or hail but impossible to walk on, lethal to drive on and invisible, apart from a tell-tale shininess if you know what to look for.

The place to see most easily is in the trees – cue another arty photograph – because each twig on every branch develops a coating of ice. Imagine dipping a tree in molten glass and upending it back in the ground, allowing the glass to set. I know I've gone all lyrical again but I've never seen anything quite so magnificently strange. For a day Kitchener looked like a computer generated idea for a planet made of glass. I could imagine hearing tinkly footsteps as little glass people appeared from their glassy woodland glen. And there is a sort of sound to be heard when you're outside. Very faint, it's a sort of cross between a rustle and a tinkle. It's the sound of ice forming. Pretty.

The freezing rain delayed our trip to the snow dump by a day or two but we got there in the end. No-one can understand why we should want to but for us it was a must. It's only a heap of snow with several bulldozers on top but when I say heap of snow I mean one that has room for several bulldozers on top. I think the fascination lies in the fact that it exists at all. Rather like the leaf hoover. It's obvious when you think about it that there would need to be such an amenity but I'd never have generated the idea in my head just by imagining living here.

No-one understands most of the things we want to go and see, recommendations come thick and fast:

'When you're in Toronto you must see Casa Loma, it's a castle!'

'Do go to Ottawa and see the parliament buildings.'

'Fergus is very pretty, it's an old village.'

We say thank you politely each time and make a mental note not to bother. It's a little like telling someone who lives in the Rockies to be sure and take in the Ben Nevis Race when they visit the UK. People who know us well are beginning to understand that we have history at home but we don't have geology or wildlife. They can see that waterfalls and beaver dams might be more appealing than castles but their eyes glaze over when I mention snow dumps.

* * *

Zuscha has a cold. A drippy snivelly miserable cold. She has a permanent dewdrop on the end of her nose and spends her time wandering from room to room saying 'oh by dose'. I follow her about like an obedient puppy with box of tissues but the connection is a little beyond her. She's stopped singing and has been getting cross with the cats. She must be feeling awful. She isn't up to the link between feeling ill and taking to bed, which must be a horrible experience. I'm running out of ideas and I think I'm getting the cold.

We've met the new neighbours by the way, I did manage to keep Zuschy out of the undergrowth for long enough for the house to sell in the end. I've been meaning to pop next door and say 'hi' since they moved in but Zuscha beat me to it. Although I'm not sure that attacking their flower pots with a broom somewhat in the manner of Don Quixote is the best way to make friends. They were very nice about it.

I wasn't sure what to do next. I think the Canadian way would be to take a home-baked pie round but baking isn't terribly practical in such a muddy kitchen so I decided to make do with a friendly explanatory visit. And it finally happened. I'm surprised it's taken so long, I really am. Someone has asked me at last if I've met a Royal. Fortunately I was able to oblige since I once protected the Queen from certain death at a farming exhibition in Hyde Park. Well, all I did was sit in my ambulance really but had mortality threatened I'd have leapt into action almost as though I'm not a raving republican. Neighbour suitably impressed. Clearly I am a proper Brit with adequate curiosity value. I then blew the image completely by declining a cup of tea in favour of coffee.

The Firm are very popular in this part of ex-colony, which is why I can rely on *The Record* to keep me up to date with important developments at home. I understand the Queen Mother has had a nosebleed.

My nose is definitely starting to dribble. I made the mistake of venturing out tissueless. A small omission but it led to one those delightful encounters that make this country such fun. I popped into a garage to fill the car with petrol. It occurred to me while paying in the kiosk thingy, that pocket-sized packets of hankies often lurk among the Mars Bars and air-fresheners. I asked the girl behind the counter if they sold tissues. 'No we don't' she said, 'but I've got a box here, take as many as you like.' She put the box on the counter while swiping my debit card. This little act of kindness bowled me over. She's from Newfoundland, this angel in PetroCanada employee form, and she moved here with her parents as a child. She likes Kitchener but doesn't like jokes about Newfies, who are Canada's equivalent of the Irish, joke-wise.

I wish I'd had the presence of mind to ask her name. She deserves to be immortalised in print, along with the wonderful waitress from *Gatto's*, even if my mother is the only person who'll read about her.

Ben is poorly too. Probably flu but he keeps waking up feeling dizzy. He has a slightly dodgy health history so it was off to the clinic for a fret and a worry. 'Probably flu' said the doc, 'but we'll requisition all the tests anyway.' I had arrived in battleaxe mode. I'm used to hammering desks and shouting 'I may or may not be a neurotic first-time Mum but I want it tested and I'm not budging until you sign the form' before getting anything done. So for the second time in a week I'd like to immortalise a Canadian who's just doing their job. Name? Sorry, forgot.

Just so I don't appear to be viewing the world through maple syrup tinted specs I'm going to have a moan now. I've had a spot of trouble with the car. Well, when I say a spot of trouble what I mean is a lot of inconvenience and expense as a result of my own pea-brained stupidity. We are driving around in a shiny new status symbol of a rental car just now. Not a normal state of affairs, our battered old wreck is in for a post-mortem and Pat decided to rent some transport to tide us over so that Zuscha can still go out for coffee. Ben managed to apply a huge scratch along three panels of said shiny effort with his bike.

When I came back out of orbit and stopped shouting I had a little panic and then decided to scoot around and get a few estimates for the damage before 'fessing up' to Pat and/ or rental company. I rang a little local place and explained my dilemma. They were happy to oblige so I terminated the phone call with a jolly 'see you in ten minutes then' and jumped in the car, keen to get the whole nasty business over with.

Carolyn Steele

I didn't get there that day. I had a road accident on the way. More damage on nice posh rental car. Not a lot, just a broken indicator light and a bent bumper, it wouldn't have shown up on our usual wreck of course. In fact Ben could have carved his initials on our usual wreck and no-one would have been any the wiser. However, I'm in Canada so it has to be reported to the police, presumably because they're bored.

The other car escaped unscathed for goodness sake but it still has to be reported. Which makes it an insurance job, despite the minimal damage. There's a swanky new Collision Reporting Centre at the police headquarters where you take all your paperwork. They take photographs too. Of a bumped bumper. I am getting grumpy. This country needs a few more hardened villains.

* * *

We've had an interesting spot of Pavlovian conditioning in the house. Zuscha's routine infusions have come round again. One of the cats, Misha The Smaller, usually the trouble-maker, has taken to swinging on the plastic tubing. I began to delay putting down cat food until the nurse turned up so as to distract from the obvious delights of intravenous gymnastics. Within three days, young Misha would clock the arrival of nurse plus infusion gear and make off to sit by the dinner bowl. I know I read all the required texts as a psychology undergrad about a hundred years ago but I've never seen it in action before. Clearly the cat is a good doggie after all.

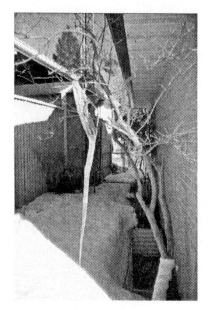

Arty stilettos

FOURTEEN

A slight technical hitch

We can all sleep again. The school talent show has been and gone and I for one am most relieved. I got into my usual state but Ben's performance was flawless as ever. He was a little disappointed with the audience response though which led us to have a long and deep discussion on the vagaries of international entertainment, a surreal experience with a ten-year-old. He felt, not unreasonably, that it couldn't have been up to his usual barnstorming audience-in-the-palm-of his-hand standard because the giggling had been a little muted. Everyone made complimentary comments afterwards but still, something felt different.

Canadian humour is generally a lot less subversive than we're used to. There's a political satire on the TV that actually runs a warning along the lines of *some of you may not share our sense of humour because it's satirical*. I find the warning a lot funnier than the show but that's not the point. We decided we'd discovered that a school full of Canadian kids felt less than comfortable with the kind of slightly naughty silliness we take for granted at home. I asked Ben which act had brought the house down. It was the cute toddler dressed in red and white who waved a Canadian flag and sang an excruciating song about how nice it is to live in Canada. 'That's the answer then' I said, suddenly inspired, 'next time we'll find a way for you to produce a Canadian flag out of the headmaster's ear.' We had a good laugh and he feels better now.

Which is more than the car does. The saga continues. I finally made it to the repair centre the following day. 'That was a long ten minutes' quipped a friendly voice from under a car when it heard my accent. 'The longest ten minutes of my life' quoth I, 'let me tell you about it.' When the assembled car people had finished laughing he supplied the punchline. 'This scratch would have polished right out for twenty-five bucks.'

Yes, if I hadn't been in such a state about it that could easily have been the end of the story. The extra mauling I managed to give the bumper will cost a little more. And because this is Canada and it had to be reported to the police and go through the insurance company I need three estimates. What do these people do all day? I will never voluntarily drive another rental car as long as I live. The stress is indescribable. Give me life and death any day.

And speaking of life and death, an interesting court case has hit the headlines this week. There is a byelaw in the town of Blue Mountain, Ontario that forbids noise pollution. We have a similar thing back home to prevent all night parties and outlandish stereos etc. Blue Mountain is a more genteel establishment however (a ski resort, you will recall, if you have been taking notes) so the nuisance decibel level is a tad lower. Some chap is suing his neighbour for having a Canadian flag outside his house that flaps too loudly in the wind. I'm not sure whose side I am on here.

While I'm trawling the paper for transcultural charm, I ought to fill you in on the latest with Williegate – taking the cookie these days, biscuits are scones. Several charitable collections are under way in the memory of our favourite ex-rodent. Not only individual contributions to the Ontario Veterinary College but a trust fund in his name for the Children's Wish Foundation. It started as a workplace gag but so many people put their hands in their pockets that the money ended up having to go somewhere. Gobsmacked twice in a week.

I had a load of photos back this week. Some of my arty-fartier shots haven't materialised. I clearly need a driving lesson on my camera. As well as – oh never mind. The weird and wonderful icicles have survived but the glass trees will have to remain a fanciful description. Ditto the snow dump, although I do have a super pic of the road sign that says Snow Dump. I'm very proud of it. Not so sure about the one of me celebrating turning forty-two by looking as dippy as possible on a child's toboggan. Ben says it's 'pretty neat'. I still hate that word.

A worrying thing has happened. Ben and I went out for supper. Not perturbing in itself, we do it a lot but this occasion was the first on which we have ever both completely cleared our plates. We ate it all, mountain of pasta, trough full of salad and the garlic bread. In our defence we had finally found the winning meatball but it's still a worry. Especially since I then found myself surveying the dessert menu as though I could find a corner for a spot of pud. I was wrong of course but even contemplating such folly wouldn't have happened when we first arrived. Now our appetites are trained to transatlantic standards we are clearly destined to balloon to enormous size. The odd bout of energetic skating is unlikely to save us.

I think half our trouble is a delight with sitting in the eateries themselves. We are getting used to feeling unintimidated and it seems to be in restaurants that we unwind properly and start to talk. Because one sits about waiting for things I suppose. Not only do we search for the finest meatball, we ponder all the other mysteries of life this trip is unearthing for us too. For instance, we've put our minds recently to the puzzling phrase *Nous ne servons que de Heinz*. I am used to pointless translation in bilingual countries to a certain extent. Anyone who has driven much in Wales and has marvelled at road signs that say the same thing twice if the place name happens to be spelt the same in English and Welsh would be quite at home with most of the signs here. I actually find Canadian postal vans rather endearing, still reading 'MAIL POSTE' along the side and wondering for a second which is the English.

It's the absolute necessity to translate catchphrases on packaging that has me baffled. Particularly when the translation is neither a catchphrase or a translation. It is in restaurants that one reads the items on bottle and jar labels isn't it? Every Heinz Tomato Ketchup bottle on every table in every restaurant in town sports the natty little jingle *We serve no other Keinz*; in French *Nous ne servons que du Heinz*. Now if my faltering French can be trusted this means *We don't serve anything that isn't Heinz*. It's not a pun, it's not a rhyme, it's not a direct translation, what is it? I'll tell you what it is, it's silly. (And what's more, Aero is not only *Big on Bubbles* but *Les bulles, on s'y connait!* as well. What's the French for silly?)

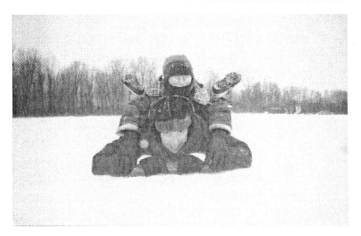

Forty-two

Zuscha has paid a visit to hospital. Another bit of a worry. For no apparent reason her blood sugar shot through the roof yesterday morning. And kept on rising. The only unusual occurrence had been the accidental consumption of a daffodil bulb in the night, which I was expecting to produce more in the line of vomiting and diarrhoea than hyperglycaemia but what do I know? I decided to do the decent thing and invade the local Emergency Room.

It was an entertaining afternoon. For the entire department. May I remind you that Zuscha is extremely deaf? Just for those of you not taking notes. The nice nurse asked us for a urine sample and handed me a bowl. 'You must be joking' I whimpered. But sadly not. My increasingly inventive attempts to persuade Zuscha, at the top of my voice, to comprehend what it was we had to do in the bowl were much enjoyed by staff and patients alike. In desperation I tried pleading that it would be quicker to wait for her to have an accident and then squeeze out the knickers but everyone missed the point, I'd used the wrong word. They took a blood sample in the end, probably still wondering where the knickers were.

The doctor asked what had alerted me to the problem.

'Well, she started to look a bit ropy after breakfast...' I began.

'Ropy' she said, 'I like that, can I use it? What does it mean?' Well what does ropy mean? I know what I mean and I expect you know what I mean but try to define it. I failed. The doctor grinned. Then Zuscha saved the day by nose-diving into my handbag, scattering the contents across the floor and falling upon Ben's copy of *The Beano* – thoughtfully sent from home for us by a chum – and reading it to us both. Ever heard Dennis the Menace read aloud before? Neither had Kitchener's Grand River hospital.

We waited a good while. Not as long as we'd have waited in your average London casualty department I don't think but still long enough for Zuschy to be better by the time her blood was tested again. They very kindly investigated the toxicity of various garden bulbs while we were there. Apparently she'll live, it was just sugar. Did you know that daffodil bulbs are sweet to eat? They gave her some disgusting looking supper and we were released. It's reassuring to see that hospital food is grey the world over.

* * *

I was intending to muse this week about why it is that Canadians don't travel much while Australians do it all the time and Brits come to it later in life. And sometime I will, it's an interesting ponder. Events have overtaken musings however and life has become interesting. In the sense of the curse.

I have been sacked. By email. All of a sudden. Apparently I'm expensive. The new house is ready and it would appear that Ben and I are now surplus to requirements. Pat is on her way to collect Zuscha, we may remove ourselves at the end of the week.

You'll have to forgive a slight sense of humour failure here. I hadn't the least idea this was coming. In addition to being expensive I am also difficult, uncommunicative, irrational and I overreact to stress. I have been all these things since Christmas.

It's probably all true enough. Strangely, when we arrived here and got to know Pat while she was caring for Zuscha single-handedly, she seemed to me to be all of the above. Perhaps these are the naturally occurring traits of a truly burnt-out resident of Planet Alzheimer. In which case, won't it all happen again with the next person? Running this concept politely past Pat may, in retrospect, have been a mistake though. She has found someone in BC to care for Zuscha when they move, this is obviously cheaper than moving Ben and me and I can understand her trying to economise but if I'm really so many awful things, how come she entrusted her Mum to me so long?

Within twenty-four hours of the news breaking, everybody who knew us had offered to do something to help. Those with bed space offered us accommodation, those with basement space offered us storage for our things, everyone who worked with me offered a reference (even the chap who runs the lunch club Zuscha absconded from on her ill-fated dandelion binge) and the ones who couldn't do anything else booked a night to take us out for dinner to cheer us up.

My full and frank admission of all recently attributed personality defects has been cast aside for other interpretations of Pat's decision. Oddly enough several people are blaming themselves. I had mentioned being a bit apprehensive about Pat's Christmas visit and my beloved support system had promised to tell Pat how well they thought I was managing. They are now concerned that they may have inadvertently created a perceived imbalance in the wonderfulness stakes, which necessitated my removal.

Pat does like to be The Only One Who Can Cope, so it is one possible explanation. To be honest, flattering though this interpretation of events may be, I think the irrational and difficult version may be closer to the mark. Only I know quite how many times I approached breaking point after all. And you too now obviously. No time to brood however, we had the rest of our adventure to plot. I could put off naval-gazing with regard to my personal failings but I couldn't put off a disappointed little boy.

We spent a day getting over the shock and then began making our plans around the things people wanted to do for us. I gave Ben the choice of helping to decide what happened next or leaving it to me. He opted to join in the thinking so after a rapid interview with an immigration advisor we listed our options.

Under the terms of my visa I'd be allowed to stay on and look for similar work if I wished, so this left us with three alternatives. We could come home and get back to normal, we could stay with chums in Kitchener and look for another live-in job or we could store our things in Holly's basement, fly out to the West Coast anyway and look for work there. This was the clear winner. Even if no job materialised, Ben would finally get to see a banana slug out west. I have a feeling that once he's crossed banana slugs and whales off the list he'll go home relatively content.

More help happened. Theresa has a sister in Vancouver who will be more than happy to meet us off the plane, put us up until we get ourselves sorted and show us around. She will do this because her sister is fond of us. Have I mentioned lately how nice Canadians are? I discussed the germinating scheme with an email pen pal on Vancouver Island and had jobcentre information by return. And offers of hospitality and personalised tour guide services.

Mother asked me why we didn't just call it an exciting year and come home. How could I possibly let all these people down? They want Ben to see his slug, the least we can do is give it a try. Canada has to be the best country in the world to find yourself in trouble in.

The final plan involves blowing some cleverly squirreled away air miles on leg two of The Great Canadian Adventure. We will fly to Vancouver, recover from our recent angst and get our BC sea legs chez Theresa's sister Sharon, then hop on a ferry to Victoria and jobhunt courtesy of a nice-sounding chap called Joe. That way Ben gets to live for a while on An Island. Possibly a short while but you never know eh?

My last week with Zuschy was too busy for musings of the poignant kind. We would be allowed to stay on for a short while if we needed time to find a new home but I was still out of a job, very upset and in fear of my opinions by then. Staying on while the house was packed up around us wasn't an emotional option, although I would hate to give the impression that Pat threw a child out on the street. By the time she returned we were organised. Everything we could possibly leave behind was boxed, inventoried and stored in Holly's basement. I can just ship it all home if need be. The rest we'll lug about until we find a new place to collect junk in. How can two people (one small) acquire so much stuff in a year?

In what seemed like no time at all we were on the plane. Ben visited the pilot as usual. The stewardess asked me if I'd like to visit the flight deck too.

'I thought only little boys got to do that.'

'Oh no, big kids can go along too.'

Ben generally does a good line in charming pilots. This one asked us where we lived. We looked at each other and thought hard. 'Nowhere really.'

FIFTEEN

Funky

I can now report that Theresa's sister Sharon has the most wonderful face I have ever seen. By which I mean that I have never been happier to clap eyes on anyone in my life. She was easy to spot, the only Crystal Tipps in the arrival lounge with Theresa's grin thrown in, a familiar stranger. Just what you need when there is no word for the distance between what you feel and pathetic adjectives like *exhausted*. The last week had drained the pair of us, I'd thought that organising to leave England in two months was stressful but arranging the leaving of Ontario in a week left us with something similar to jet lag.

For some reason that made sense at the time we had a flight involving a three hour connection in Calgary. There was nothing to do except eat fries – fortunately the Canadian type which are crisp enough to use to prop your eyes open – and think a little too much. We were both watching the shine come off our sparkly, clever adventure, so to be met at the airport, driven home and put to bed by the BC chapter of our adopted family was inexpressibly comforting. We slept for a very long time. And then some more. I think we ate a bit now and again between sleeps. It would appear that a year of broken nights can leave one a little tired. After a bit more sleep we thought we were fine so we arranged to move on, with many plans to reconvene as soon as I found a job. One day I'd like to make Sharon's acquaintance properly. Another addition to the list of people to whom we owe a good deal of hospitality.

It was a bit Wednesdayish when we said good-bye (and a hundred thank-yous) to Sharon and set off to seek our fortunes on An Island. We hadn't seen a great deal of Vancouver between sleeps, so all I can tell you so far is that every other shop sells something oriental and the bus station has a disconcertingly ornate ceiling. Not just a latticework of cornices and curlicues but colours and patterns and everything. I'm not a connoisseur of bus stations so there may be many such imposing temples to the travel muse for all I know but it took me a while to square the colonial elegance with catching a bus. Even the one which was going to convey us and our luggage on and off the ferry to Vancouver Island and deposit us in downtown Victoria, a few blocks from our temporary new home, the youth hostel.

Hostelling had seemed like a good idea from K/W when I booked us in but neither of us had tried it before, so although it was the only sensible way to stretch our remaining money I have to be honest and confess that neither of us fancied the idea of dormitory life too much. We oohed and ahhed a suitable amount on the ferry and congratulated ourselves regularly that this was More Like Real Travelling; but neither of us quite defeated the queasy undertone that accompanies realising that you are now performing entirely without the aid of a safety net.

The hostel, when we found it, was a relatively pleasant surprise. Friendly, clean, warm, a TV room for Ben, a kitchen for me, power sockets for laptopping (hooray) and best of all, a little bedroom all to ourselves. This last was the result of much rearranging by the hostel staff because they thought it would be nicer for Ben and I am eternally grateful. Have I mentioned recently how nice Canadians are?

Just when I realised our accommodation was going to be fine – shortly after finding Ben being taught to play pool by an Australian with hairy knees – I began to have serious doubts about my chances of getting another job. Despite all the safety-net related unease, nothing had gone wrong so far which meant that the inevitable glitch was still to come. An absence of work was the only glitch left and things weren't looking promising. All the job agencies seemed to work on the 'leave a message and we'll ring you back' system and the big disadvantage of hostel life is that they can't. I went through a fortune in quarters trying to catch human beings to talk to and was beginning to lose the irrepressible sense of optimism that got this mad jaunt off the ground in the first place. Still, with a book to finish there was only one thing for it, hit town and see as much as we could anyway.

If Vancouver is oriental, Victoria is, well, *funky*. No other word quite fits sitting in the market square surrounded by art galleries, Guatemalan bead emporia and organic falafel outlets. I don't know if it's possible to Feng Shui a pedestrian precinct but if it can be done then it will have been. As I sat in the square scribbling a few notes about the restful tinkly music, a small but lively scuffle spilled out from the *Avalon Metaphysical Centre*. A frank exchange of views along the lines of 'you have abandoned the spirit, your store is forever evil' was quickly and quietly dealt with by a couple of market square security guards, clearly used to metaphysical fisticuffs. Yeah, funky.

The harbour is almost as surreal. Imposing colonial buildings, mountainy backdrop and loads of tiny ferries chugging around and across each other's paths to get from one side of the harbour to the other, rather like an aquatic Morris dance. Another nice place to sit and chill, as long as you don't mind being buzzed by seaplanes. In Ontario you hang out by the way, in British Columbia you chill. I know this courtesy of my ex-email pal Joe, who is rapidly becoming tour guide, cook, escort, all-round source of information and general saviour. Ben's not much of a one for hanging or chilling but Joe has found him a beach where lumps of jade lurk among the pebbles and driftwood washed in by the Pacific. Sadly it's pretty low grade stuff so I won't be putting him to work polishing and selling it on street corners just yet but jade it is. He has a goodly haul already and is happily scouring the shops for a second hand stone-tumbling machine with his sights set on a career in jewellery-making.

Meanwhile I have learned the quickest way to get the hang of a new town, you need to find out which newspapers to read. Kitchener was easy, *The Record* was the only option but Victoria, being a great deal more cosmopolitan, has a choice of organ. I now know that the *Times Colonist* is the one for job ads, second-hand bikes and reactionary editorial. The *Monday Magazine* – which comes out on Thursday, I love that – is the place for arty listings, quirky stories and opportunities to volunteer in women's refuges. The *Victoria News* is, well, a bit boring actually. (How do I know all this? Joe, natch.) Armed with my new expertise I set about trying to invent the next new life for us. There isn't a lot of work about if you stick to jobcentres and agencies but the *Times* classifieds looked more hopeful. Four applications in the post and I didn't feel quite so much as though we were wasting our time. I unwound enough to do a little proper sightseeing.

And sightseeing is what one does here, it's what Victoria is for. Tourism has been the main industry since they built Vancouver and forgot to extend the railway. Before that it was opium, of which more later. I'll gloss over the replica of Anne Hathaway's cottage and other such nonsense designed to con the Yanks into thinking they're on a day trip to England and move straight to the wonderful Bug Zoo. For the princely sum of ten bucks you get to see a lot of insects. Well, Ben likes such things so in we went.

Your ten bucks includes the undivided attention of an entomology student for as long as you wish to devise silly questions. They love their bugs. They want you to love them too and I have to admit we very nearly did. I'm not keen on bugs as such but am completely sold on anywhere that provides you with an enthusiastic expert of your own for less than the cost of a pizza. I might even go back a second time.

Unlike the Royal British Columbia Museum. It's terribly good, worthy displays that walk you through stories of native legend, a fake gold mine to keep the kids quiet until they lose the feeling in their hands panning in cold water and an awful lot of totem poles. Now I know totem poles are fantastic pieces of work and very meaningful and all that but one or two would have been sufficient for me. Ben enjoyed it well enough and panned for gold until his fingers went blue but on the whole I preferred the superb chips in the cafe afterwards. To be fair, my usual antipathy to museums may have been to blame, I'm sure it's a fine example of the genre really but if you ever find yourself there make sure to try the chips.

One thing is clear, I haven't done enough chilling yet. I'd rather be sitting by the water than doing museums and I think I've found the ideal place to do it. We jumped on a bus the other day in search of a place that advertised amazingly cheap accommodation. The hostel may be fun but it's noisy. Neither of us has been getting much rest and we fancied moving on. Besides, access to a telephone might significantly enhance my employment prospects. The bus was bound for a little place called Sooke, not far from Victoria, just a few kilometres along the coast and utterly magical. New combinations of mountains, forests and sea opened up each time the bus rounded another corner and by the time we alighted at the *Save-On Gas* station we were open-mouthed that you could go anywhere so dramatic on anything as ordinary as a bus.

We found our new home a stone's throw from the bus stop in the most delightful spot I have ever seen. It's a throw of the same stone in the other direction to the sea and the house is set in a bit of forest, with a spectacular view of the Olympic Mountains across the water in the States. It smells green. For the same amount of money as we are spending at the hostel, a nice couple (who appear to have taken to us) would like to feed us three meals a day, with packed lunches if the mood takes us to go out.

I've booked for a month and bought a bicycle. Well, it's also a stone's throw (same stone) from the Galloping Goose cycle network, which takes you and your bike through spectacular bits of island along the route of an old railway line. It is therefore considerably flattish and perfect for cycling. The Galloping Goose was once the train.

The idea is to call my month in Sooke a holiday. Not a haring-about-seeing-and-doing-it-all holiday. More of a sitting-by-the-Pacific-and-contemplating-the-mountains sort of thing. I've decided I've earned it. If a job hasn't materialised in a month's time, I'll…well…sit and think some more probably. This place sort of gets you that way. It's full of people who drifted by and never quite got around to doing anything about moving on. Originally one blamed the opium dens, now it's a proud tradition.

But then we had to do it, the temptation was too much. Much as we needed our retreat by the sea, we were seduced by the idea of one more bit of haring-about-seeing-and-doing-it-all before the big rest. I'm not much of a camper generally but the hostel advertised a group camping trip that happened to include all our Vancouver Island must-dos in three days. I signed up in a moment of weakness. Joe cast a jaundiced eye at the sky when I mentioned it. 'I'll have a hot meal waiting when you get back.' Mary would approve.

Does Joe know everything? Probably. It rained. It was freezing. It snowed a bit. It was also the greatest fun imaginable. Two Aussies, a Dane, two Brits and three Canadians hiked in rain forests, picnicked by waterfalls, baked local salmon on beach fires and watched the sun go down over the mighty Pacific. I'm not being soppily poetic here, those waves are enormous. Our guide – the fabulous Sindy, who thinks of everything – told us horrifying stories of rogue waves which could wash you away out to sea, never to be seen again. This not just for Ben's benefit, he was relatively sensible compared to the macho Canadian with a girlfriend to impress who regularly terrified us all with his dopey rock-climbing exploits. The more rattled Sindy became with regard to the group's safety, the more reckless this gentleman's behaviour.

Scientific explanations of the rogue wave phenomenon didn't work, pleading to set an example to younger members of the group didn't work, neither did shouting. He progressed from always hopping one rock nearer the surf than everyone else as we walked, to clambering over safety rails at lookout points. I can see how hard it must be to maintain a healthy respect for the elements when one's hormones are at work but poor Sindy had a hard time coping. Eventually, in a quiet moment I asked her, half in fun, whether she had ever lost someone from one of her groups. Then I understood. Yes, a chap had been swept away on his honeymoon. No-one's fault, a rogue, rogue wave which curled a tongue around the group as they stood what should have been a safe distance from the shoreline. I began to see why she might twitch a little at showing-off time.

The hormones were flying in both directions for our pet Canadian couple. She, also keen to impress and clearly of the opinion that her long blonde hair was her most arresting feature, had an interesting habit of leaping in front of every camera anyone raised to photograph a scenic spot and elaborately combing her locks in front of it. No-one asked her not to. It was such an odd phenomenon that none of us quite realised it would keep on happening until it happened again. And then it was too late.

We camped near enough to the beach to be able to hear the ocean during the night. The sound will stay with me forever. Not quite thunder but nearer to it than anything else. I am running out of superlatives. Sindy taught us to put up the tents, built the fire and cooked our supper. When we woke in the morning, Sindy was making pancakes and coffee. Sindy is superwoman.

We went whale watching. Grey whales, we had the wrong season for Orcas which was a shame, Ben adopted an Orca from a local pod a couple of years ago. It would have been fun to give it a photo of us and buy it some shoes. We bobbed about in a boat that didn't feel that tiny in the harbour and waited. Just us and the eagles. As we sat we'd see spouts of water here and there. We began to see the pattern: dive deep for food, ten, maybe fifteen minutes then back to the surface for a spout or two. Then an arch of the back, one last blow, a flip of the tail and back to the bottom amid the whirring of a dozen cameras. Even our pet macho man was awed into silence. Ben's face was indescribable. As was the strange yearning we all had to be a whale. To be so graceful and beautiful and peaceful. Now I am getting soppily poetic. It was quite something anyway.

Our only disappointment throughout the trip was the total absence of banana slugs. We hiked through Cathedral Grove – their regular hideout – but it's unseasonably cold this year (tell me about it) and the slugs aren't about yet.

We'll just have to go back someday. I did get some wonderful photographs of trees though. Trees too enormous and ancient to be imaginable unless you've experienced being dwarfed by them. You can tell how big they are because there's this tiny blonde person combing her hair in front of each one.

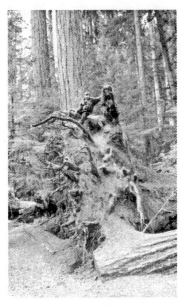

Blonde-free tree

With the photographic bug re-established I took my camera around Victoria on our return, majoring on Chinatown. Victoria has the oldest Chinatown in North America, I never knew that. But then I've only just twigged why this area is so Oriental. It's on the Pacific. Yes I know I've just spent three days camping by the stuff but I only looked at a globe properly this week. Directly across the mighty thunderous one we find (somewhat belatedly) Japan, Hawaii, China, The Philippines. As Joe has patiently explained to me, there's a blooming great range of mountains between the West Coast and the rest of the continent of North America, anyone from the Pacific Rim who heads east hits the coast of BC first and tends to stay. British Columbians consider themselves a Pacific nation. They'd witter about separation *a la* Quebec if they weren't too busy chilling.

Victoria appears to have been built on the twin pillars of colonial affectation and opium. In 1889 there were over a dozen opium factories here. It all started perfectly legally in 1886 when an estimable gent called Lem Chung paid 250 dollars for a licence to sell the stuff. By the time Canada followed the States into thinking this was a Bad Thing in 1908 business was booming. So it went sort of officially underground and everyone was relatively happy. There was a brief flurry of disapproval in 1884, mainly due to concern that Chinese immigrants would work for less than locals – there's a remarkably intricate salmon gutting machine in the Royal British Columbia Museum by the way, engraved with the name *Mechanical Chink* – anyway, a Commission on Chinese Immigration visited the opium dens on a tut-tutting tour and found some (shock, horror) white people there, including a famous prostitute called Emily Wharton. She assured them that she'd been smoking the stuff for years and considered it far less harmful than alcohol. So they decided it was probably OK after all and that was that.

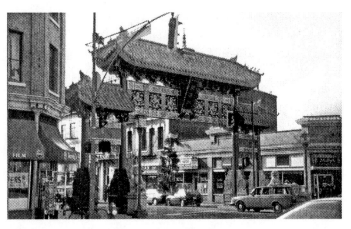

Chinatown...the front

Chinatown now stands cheek by jowl with all the architectural splendour of an otherwise Victorian showpiece... the Masonic Library in one street and in the next, tiny shops that go back and back getting ever smaller till they taper off into more of an alley than a building. Behind the tiny shop/alleys, derelict little warehouses face onto tiny squares, their windows covered with iron bars. This was the Forbidden City. These were the opium dens. The bars at the windows look solid enough but they moved if you had the knack. That's how you disappeared.

Joe muttered darkly about getting us a peek behind the scenes and schmoozed a friendly shopkeeper; we were permitted to sneak out the back and gaze in awe at ex-forbiddendom. I took a photo. It's very ordinary.

We left the hostel a little regretfully in the end. It had only been two weeks but we seemed to have made a lot of friends. Ben's Australian friend left a day or two ahead of us and gave me the remains of his Vegemite. Isn't that nice? It's an odd bond, yeast extract. Only Brits and Aussies share it. All other nationalities sniff the stuff suspiciously, wrinkle their noses a lot and don't get the point of the flavour. I think you need to have been brought up with the stuff to get it. I have the same trouble with root beer.

Digressing slightly here, I shared my London home with a refugee from Bosnia a few years ago, during the height of the ethnic cleansing. All her friends passed through my kitchen at some time or other, including a girl from Croatia who'd been an *au pair* in England when the war first started and got stuck here as a result. Yes, she'd adjusted to life here very well she told me and her English had greatly improved but there was one thing she absolutely couldn't learn to cope with. Well I had to enquire. It was Marmite.

Back to Sooke, or more correctly Sasseenos, which is just before you get to Sooke, can a village have a suburb? Sasseenos is Salish Indian for *sunny land sloping gently up from the sea*. I read that on a heritage notice along the cycle trail. It wasn't easy tearing my eyes away from the backdrop of foresty, mountainy stuff but since someone had gone to the trouble of providing me with a nugget of information on a heritage notice it would have been churlish not to read it.

I've never lived in the country before. Not proper countryside country where the buses are rare. If you miss one, it's an hour-and-a-half before the next. That's serious countryside in my book. Fortunately the bus timetable is pretty accurate, although I suppose it would be difficult for it not to be, so long as you remember that they all turn up five minutes early. Usually. But sometimes it's five minutes late. I forgot to allow the five minutes this morning. We stood for a while cursing our forgetfulness, then turned to pop home for a cuppa before the next bus of the day. Naturally the bus flew by just as we rounded the corner out of sight. Our hosts were most impressed. 'Nobody's missed the bus quite like that before.'

Our hosts (who do have names but we took to calling them Hinge and Bracket so early in our stay that they will remain so-called to us forever) seem fond of us but are proving to be rather trying company. I feel I should be learning from the political opinions Hinge spouts over the newspapers after meals but my attention is drawn inexorably to Bracket, twitching with the effort of finding a chink in the conversation to change the subject. Her preferred topics are the habits of neighbours, especially their tendency to train their pets to annoy her; and dark intimations of the nefarious doings of sundry previous boarders. Her specialist subject, once Hinge has taken their irrepressibly irritable dog for a walk though, is Hinge and his shortcomings. Bracket can't walk the dog owing to a tendency to topple over if anything appears too suddenly in her peripheral vision. One of the house rules involves not inadvertently creeping up on Bracket. I think there are probably going to be other house rules.

Occasionally they call a truce for long enough to be very good company and I will treasure their egg story for ever. It's another travelling food tale. Stopping at a roadside eatery for breakfast one day, they were pleased to note that the establishment served *eggs any style*. Hinge ordered a fried egg, Bracket a poached one. The waitress looked a little perplexed. She disappeared into the kitchen and returned most apologetic, 'I'm sorry, we don't have poached eggs, we just have eggs any style.'

* * *

Ben has started another new school. A nerve-wracking enough enterprise at the best of times but this time round we have had to learn about the School Bus. Which is not the same as an ordinary bus. School buses are such a highly revered institution that someone not quite understanding how the system works is beyond the ken of any but the most open-minded Canadian. I'm back to square one stupid-question-wise and we got it all wrong on the first day but we're seasoned hands now. We know where to pick it up in the morning, where to expect it to drop Ben off in the afternoon and where to find the number to check it's the right bus. And I'm going to tell you about a great idea. I was impressed when I read it, a lifetime ago, mugging up on Canadian rules of the road before we left England. I've been doing it like a good Canadian driver since I arrived but it's only just re-entered my consciousness as a concept, presumably because my kid's involved.

It's an offence to drive past a school bus that's loading or unloading children. The buses sport big red flashing lights that go on when they pull in to deal with their cargo and traffic has to stop in both directions until the lights cease. There are few more heinous crimes on a Canadian road than passing a school bus. Children hop off and cross the road in perfect safety. Isn't that neat?

Oh no, another quarter in the Neat Box.

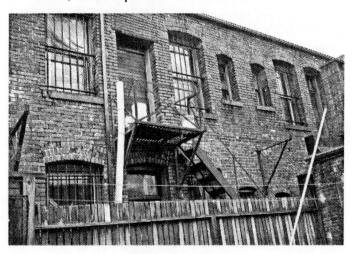

Chinatown…the back

SIXTEEN

Small mysteries

A faintly alarming form has come home from school for my attention. It's the Emergency Preparedness Plan and Release Form. It details arrangements to be made in the event of a major seismic event. They mean an earthquake. It explains how the children will be evacuated from buildings and mustered on the playing field and how they will only be released into the care of people detailed on our forms. In addition to the usual information about designated alternative caregivers, we must supply the phone number of someone off the island, preferably on a cell phone, who can take messages when all the landlines are down. We must send our children to school with a sealed bottle of water by way of emergency provisions. There is also a list of ways you may be able to help when it happens; if you are a carpenter or engineer for example, or a radio ham or an owner of many tents. I've offered my vast first aid expertise.

It makes an interesting contrast to the release form his Ontario school sent home, that was for ice storms and buses stuck in snowdrifts. We've moved from serious weather to serious geography. Eager for more earthquake advice, I devoured the information page in our local telephone directory. There is another emergency kit to collect. We need a battery-operated radio, a good flashlight and enough bottled water, non-perishable food and spare batteries for three days. The best place to stand, if you can't get out of the house, is in a doorway. It's a good idea to know how to turn off your gas supply and a bad idea to hang pictures over the bed.

Suddenly I'm not so sure about staying here. 'It's OK' everyone says, 'they're very rare, we just have to be prepared because the Pacific Basin is an official earthquake zone.' Phew. 'And tsunamis are pretty rare too, although you'd be in trouble living that near the beach if we get one.' Tsunamis? Yes, another natural disaster to worry about. A tsunami is a tidal wave, I didn't know that. They're generated by earthquakes under the sea. An earthquake anywhere in the Pacific Basin can cause a tsunami all over our house. The telephone book information page helpfully advises 'do not go to the beach to watch.' And just as well, I might have done so but I won't now I've been told not to. How very exotic.

I have moved pictures and stocked up on batteries and water. Ben takes his earthquake supplies to school every day and is now fully conversant with earthquake drill. I wish I'd had earthquake drill at school, it sounds so much more fun than the fire variety, you have to clamber under your desk and stay there until the teacher says the earthquake is over. Then you stay under your desk and count to sixty for aftershocks. Then you head for the great outdoors. The big geography lesson just got bigger.

And what, you may ask, have I been doing with my days as Ben masters basic survival on the playing fields? Well I've had a spot more trouble with buses. It's the getting off you see. At home, when you stand by the door of a bus and it pulls into a stop, the doors open with a nice pfoosh sound, regardless of whether or not you are paying attention. The driver does it. Here, you stand gormlessly about until you realise that the driver isn't going to do it and then start looking for instructions. Well I do. And, being Canadians, all the other people on the bus sit quietly waiting for you to work it out.

I thought I had the whole business sussed until this afternoon. The nice brand-new low-floor buses – with bike racks on the front, what a fab idea that is – have huge yellow vertical handles on the doors. They say in big letters 'touch bar to open'. This isn't strictly accurate. If you put a finger gingerly on the yellow bit to see what happens, nothing happens. You have to push ever so slightly in the right direction to open. Not too hard mind, or you're still pushing when the door opens and you deposit yourself in the street at an embarrassed little run.

I got on an older type bus today. One thankfully devoid of yellow bars with instructions. So I waited for the driver to open the doors. And, being Canadian, all the other people on the bus waited politely for me to work it out. The sign for this alternative form of self-service vehicular egress is above your head. Tricky eh? 'To open door step down onto top step.' I tried it. It worked. I was so overcome with amazement I forgot to get off the bus. I stood on the top step with pride surveying my open doors. The Sooke commuters are being remarkably tolerant.

* * *

We've been dragon boat racing. Well, not exactly racing. This was more like two dragon boats full of novices splashing each other a lot. In fact it was two dragon boats full of novices splashing each other a lot. Every year you see, shortly before the start of the tourist season, Victoria opens its interesting bits to the locals. For one glorious afternoon everything is free. Including the dragon boat rides. Dragon boats are long and thin. They have a dragon's head (carved) at one end and a drummer (real) at the other. Paddled properly, by people with biceps, they are stupendously fast. With all the drumming and whatnot the races are a sufficiently oriental spectator sport to keep the harbour operating at optimal funkiness, although I do have a quibble with the person who likened it to drag racing on water. No parachutes.

We visited the Crystal Garden too on 'Be a Tourist In Your Own Town Day'. It was once the largest heated salt-water swimming pool in the British Empire. You may have known about tsunamis but I bet you didn't know that. Originally built as a glass roofed entertainment palace for Victoria's finest gentlefolk, it's a tropical garden-cum-aviary these days. I engaged unwilling-child-being-dragged-round-museum mode as usual but there were sufficient exotic orchids and cuddly, furry fruit bats to keep even me amused for a while. Neither the Dragon Boats nor the Crystal Garden offered the best free find of the day though, that honour has to go to St. Ann's Academy.

It's a nicely restored ex-convent with a suitably gold-leafed chapel (splendid ceiling). I won't bother you with when the more baroque wings were added because far more exciting is the world's smallest folly lurking in the garden. Apparently some potty priest used to creep into the grounds at night and – build stuff. So, hidden away among the trees is a little heap of rubble and scrap metal which resembles a boat. It's between two other little heaps of rubble and scrap metal which resemble – from some angles – a lighthouse and castle respectively.

Joe, who accompanied us on this and most other jaunts, has read somewhere that mystical significance of the Masonic kind could be read into these little edifices.

We walked round them in thoughtful mode, applying much imagination to the sightlines but I'm not convinced. What delighted me most was to finally find something over here that's smaller than everything over there. 'Oh in England our follies much bigger than this. In fact they're enormous.'

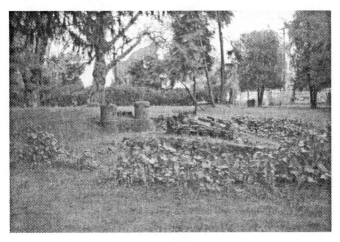

Small follies

The relentless sightseeing is a bit of a reaction to hitting a snag. Canadian Human Resources are of the opinion that I'm not entitled to seek work. In addition, whether or not my subsisting work visa (spot the jargon, nearly an expert) allows me to seek work or not, it does not entitle us to any form of medical insurance. For that we need a fresh visa. For that I need a job. But I may not be entitled to look for one, even if I take up exotic dancing. Reckon I've just found my glitch.

This news might have made for a sombre end to the week if it weren't for the continual delight provided by the *Monday Magazine*. This superlatively whimsical organ is fast turning into my favourite read ever. Not only is it possible to get a copy on Wednesday if you really know where to look – walking around with a copy of *Monday* on Wednesday instead of Thursday is the true sign of the Victoria cognoscenti – but it has a section in the small ads called *You pissed me off*.

The entries are truly splendid and endlessly fascinating. A random selection of this week's offerings includes:

> – *To the idiot who stole my coke can stereo, would you at least drop off the tapes at the James Bay Inn.*
>
> – *To the insepid* (sic) *toad who stole my bike off the back of my car: There was no sign saying 'Bicycle Buffet', you BUFFOON, and if you knew how much I loved my bike you would know how much you just screwed your own Karma.*

I am delighted by the idea of a bicycle thief screwing his own Karma, maybe he could adjust my saddle when he's finished, but even he pales into insignificance beside:

> – *The man in the blue Toyota who so rudely cut off the funeral procession on Falaise Drive on Friday April 16 at 3 PM, you should be so lucky to have that many people at your funeral.*

I can't wait to be pissed off by someone and try placing an ad. I absolutely have to find out if it's as cathartic as it appears.

By way of a break from the buses we've been for a ride on the train. Not a train I hasten to add, the train. Vancouver Island has but one and we've been on it. I developed an obsession with this train when I saw the station, a Monopoly house about the size of someone's garage sitting in the middle of a road junction. It's got flowerpots and an elaborate roof. If you look carefully, there's a railway line too. Well once you've asked 'Is that a real station?' and been told that yes it is, the train leaves once a day and the journey is spectacular, the rest is just a matter of time. The train goes about a third of the way up the east coast of the island to a little town called Courtenay. Then it comes back. At least it does on weekdays, excluding Friday when it goes up twice but only comes back once. It doesn't go up at all on Saturday, it just comes back, because it's already there. Sundays are back to normal but a bit later in the day. I hope you've got that, it's likely to be on the test.

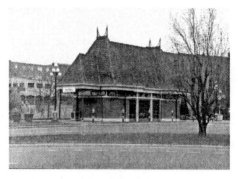

Victoria Station

'Have you got a voucher?' the lady in the station asked, when we popped in to book our trip.

'What voucher?'

'Well, there was an insert in last Sunday's *Times Colonist* with vouchers for fifty percent off train journeys, it would make a big difference to your fare. I bet there'd be one lying around in a recycle box somewhere, shall I hold on to the booking while you go and look?' Yes, I know I've said it before but here's another cheer for Canadian people just doing their job nicely. We ambled around town like a herd of marauding raccoons snuffling in people's recycle boxes and before long we had unearthed a *Times Colonist*, complete with voucher. Back at the station our lady had held the booking and was delighted for us that we had saved our fifty percent. Jaunt organised.

The only irritation was the ridiculous time we'd have to get up in the morning. No-one has adequately explained to me why one train a day must leave at quarter to eight in the morning. It's a mystery but I suppose a railway called the Esquimalt and Nanaimo is entitled to a little mystery. It certainly has a lot of bells and whistles. The journey was a perpetual series of level crossings, all of which were marked with auditory gusto. It was almost worth getting up at crack of dawn to experience the sheer joy of knowing that the occupants of every house we passed were also now awake. As the morning wore on, people started to pop out of doors to wave at the train. Not just mums and toddlers either, normal people too. Retired gents in their vegetable gardens, muscle-bound joggers, dog-walking pals, everyone waved at the train as we hooted and tooted by. I felt like one of Thomas the Tank Engine's little wooden passengers as he happily whistled a cheery 'hello' to Mrs. Kindly and all the other village worthies. Oh and the ride is spectacular too but I'm starting to use that word too much. British Columbia's like that.

Our destination, Courtenay, is famous for, well, for being the other end of the Esquimalt and Nanaimo Railway. It's a nice little town, with a goodly selection of art galleries and snow capped mountains rising majestically above the *Shopper's Drug Mart.* I took to the place in a big way when I overheard a local radio appeal for everybody in town to please keep a look out for a lost cat. Nice. Only on the west coast however would a town that tiny boast a fearfully expensive Japanese restaurant. Yup, Ben has been converted to sushi. I'm not so keen to be honest. I've always felt slightly conned by food that leaves you hungry, however pretty it may be. At least with nouvelle cuisine they bother to cook it. A bit.

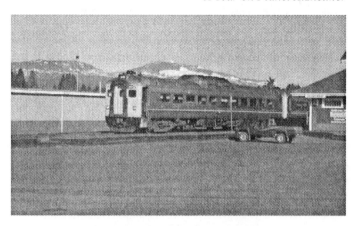

Courtenay is where the train stops

Back in Victoria the tourist season has begun overnight. The harbour has sprouted hoards of becostumed students cajoling us to eat in whichever finest restaurant in town has employed them. The costume varies from cuisine to cuisine – beefeaters begging us to eat in the finest English pub, onion bedecked Gallic charmers, the finest bistro – but the script doesn't vary. I think I preferred to saunter along the harbour front without being ambushed and told to go and eat something every time I turn a corner. By way of escape I buried myself in the library, I'd been meaning to pay it a visit for a while. It started with the dining room ceiling in the Empress Hotel. It's very ornate you see. No, I'm not off on a thesis about the British Columbian ceilings despite the apparent obsession, I just decided it was about time I delved into a little local history. People kept telling me what an interesting building the Empress was and the more they gushed the more I wanted to find out about places that didn't have elaborate ceilings. So I toddled off to the library to look up opium dens, potty folly-building priests and why the Victoria Police crest has a Masonic eye and dividers on it. Needless to say, all I could find were books about the bloody Empress. So, in a spirit of defeatism I read one. And guess what? It's a really interesting building. The aforementioned ceiling has been immortalised by Rudyard Kipling. So I guess I'm in good company.

Did you know that Winston Churchill was once served alcohol from a china teapot at the Empress? Among the delightful scandals, stories and cover-ups that this institution seems to generate I think this is my favourite. Although the love-triangle inspired murder of its architect, was pretty exciting stuff. You hear the name of Francis Rattenbury a lot here, he designed a lot of Victoria's more imposing piles. He fell from grace after divorcing his wife and marrying his mistress, who had committed the twin offences of being thirty years his junior and smoking cigarettes in public.

The happy couple moved to Bournemouth of all places where Rattenbury was eventually murdered by his young wife's even younger lover, the chauffeur. It had to be the chauffeur didn't it? Anyway he was eighteen and sentenced to hang, although after a reprieve he was released to pursue a later career of sexual assault on young boys. She was charged with murder too and then acquitted but she committed suicide anyway because she thought he was going to hang and she couldn't live without him.

Heady stuff, and there's more, but if I start on about the Empress suicides we'll never get on. People go to hotels to commit suicide all the time, I picked up countless of them in ambulance days, it's just that the Empress's clients did it with such panache. Enough already. I want to get back to Churchill's teapot because it helps to explain why it's so hard to get a drink here. Even now. British Columbia beat the States to prohibition by three years. The province was declared dry in 1917 and wet again (well, damp) by 1920 when thirsty Americans flooded over the border to try and work out how to buy a bottle of scotch. It wasn't easy. Government liquor stores (which are still here) kept civil service office hours (which they still do) and you could only make your purchase if you had about your person a personal liquor-purchase permit and were intending to consume your goods in private. Woe betide anyone opening their hard-won booze on the way home.

The Empress developed an innovative series of techniques for side-stepping the rules. Clearly taking a bottle or two to one's room was legal – that was private – although the well-tipped efforts of bellboys and porters to keep rowdy room parties supplied mightn't have been entirely kosher. Open consumption of a small sherry with dinner was right out of course because the dining room was a public place and it was illegal to consume liquor in public; however there was no law against floor length tablecloths under which could be hidden...well how could waiters possibly be expected to know what people put under their tables? Or in their teapots?

To this day it is not done to buy a beer in a bar here unless you are ordering food as well, although I'm told that a new law is in the wind to allow well-behaved establishments to set aside ten percent of their seating for the purposes of drinking rather than eating. We have found a friendly place that allows us to pretend the three of us wish to share a side of onion rings when we fancy a beer but the principle rankles a bit with this child of the land of pubs. We may not take alcohol on picnics, someone might see us and a deserted beach counts as a public place. Moreover, if by chance you find a liquor store open, you're not supposed to consume anything stronger than a Coke until you get it home. In fact, strictly speaking it is illegal to carry your bottle of wine home on the bus; public place you see and having the cork still in situ is no defence. Do I really want to live here?

While I ponder that one I'll lecture a little longer on local history, because I've unravelled another small mystery. There's a chain of up-market department stores across Canada called The Bay. Waterloo has one. It struck me as a odd name for an shop the first time I wandered in and twigged I couldn't afford anything. Now I find that they are what's left of *The Hudson's Bay Company*, without whom there is unlikely to ever have been a colony in the first place. Originally a bunch of fur traders bent on keeping the best trapping country out of the hands of Americans, it was *The Hudson's Bay Company* who sent a resourceful chap called James Douglas to Vancouver Island in 1843. He offered the local Songhee people a few hundred quid for the land Victoria stands on and built a little fort to defend the border.

The Frazer River gold rush did the rest. Suddenly Victoria was booming. It boasted the largest red light district on the west coast you know, as well as the aforementioned opium dens. Then the gold fizzled out, apart from a minor find in Sooke – not far from Ben's school, isn't that exciting? – and the town floundered a bit. When the local worthies decided to resurrect the place as a holiday destination for the rich and genteel, *The Hudson's Bay Company* opened a department store. Which is why *The Bay* is called *The Bay*. I'm so glad I know that.

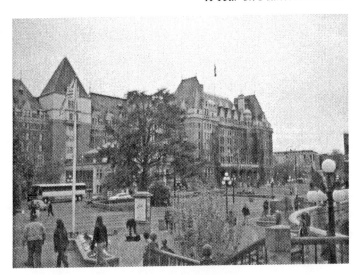

Impressive Empress

SEVENTEEN

Are we happy?

Well I'm still jobless. I found a family who would love me to care for their elderly Mum but they didn't have room for an extra Ben; I found a family who wanted me to care for their sick kiddie so much that they didn't mind an additional Ben but they can't accommodate us until some kind of property settlement is sorted out and that could take weeks. As could my appeal to Human Resources Canada. A polite man at Immigration reassured me that, yes I was entitled to look for work but no he wouldn't put it in writing for the benefit of the government department that thinks I'm not, because they don't like to encourage 'that sort of thing'. What sort of thing for goodness sake? I'm trying to look after someone's sick dependent not grow pot. Come to think of it, pot growing seems to be a more acceptable activity here than job hunting. The money will run out before the job can begin so I had to turn it down. Regretfully, they seemed very nice.

And do you know what? I'm not sure if I want to work in British Columbia anyway. There's something about the relentless laid-backness that's starting to get me down. BC may be spectacular but I fell for the Canada of baseball caps, beer bellies and neighbours who make pies. Kitchener may be one big shopping mall but I think I'm getting homesick. BC is the destination for people who would like to think they are a bit cooler than their peers. It makes for an odd atmosphere, everyone considering themselves a tad cooler, more cosmopolitan and sophisticated than the next dude. Especially when it is difficult to be truly any of these things without ever leaving a down-homey country like Canada.

Each province seems to give itself a catchphrase, 'Ontario – yours to discover' is the one we first saw on car licence plates in K/W. Out here it's 'Beautiful British Columbia' which is I think is short for 'British Columbia, too beautiful for the likes of you.'

Ben is restless too. He hasn't made friends. This is a first. We are minded to declare the place unfriendly. We cycled along our favourite bit of bike trail until we found a spot to sit and gawp at the view. Then we talked.

'Are we happy here?'

'Not really.'

'Should we stay because it's pretty?'

'Friends would be nicer.'

A couple of birds kept us company. Long legs and long beaks, that makes them eaters of fish I believe. My ornithology hasn't progressed very far. Out in the Sooke Basin a fishing boat was doing something to do with fishing. A couple of kayaks were strutting their stuff. The mountains were covered with mist, I think that means rain. We drank it in and realised that the west coast chapter of our small adventure was nearly over.

* * *

I am starting to tie up the ends, double-checking little facts at the library and taking last minute photos. We have decided to leave. And possibly just in time, the lethargy is inhalable. Now the sun's out Victoria has sprouted again. This time it's dozens of apparent street dwellers eager to convince tourists they're hungry. Since they've all appeared overnight I am tempted to infer dwellings of some sort. Sitting around somewhere nice as a career move seemed laid back and cosmopolitan when I first arrived but I'm not convinced it's a useful role model for Ben long term. We tried it. We didn't like it. I'd like to say we'd bought the T-shirt but we don't have the money. I'll miss *You pissed me off* though:

> *-To the Wicked Witch of Saxe Point whose wrath over her landscaping seems to overwhelm any compassion in her feeble soul: Thanks for destroying my Easter cheer and presents, you bitter, middle-aged old hag.*

Wouldn't you just love to know what happened in Saxe Point over Easter?

* * *

So now I'm busy again. Flight to Toronto booked and a hundred things to do. The first job is to sell Ben's bike as he has another one waiting for us in Holly's basement. This will pitch me into a major sulk, third-hand it will be worth about half what I paid for it a little over a month ago when it was second-hand. Did I spend too much on 'infrastructure' in an effort to settle? Most of it is now money down the drain. I guess if I hadn't, I'd be punishing myself for not trying hard enough to settle and wondering if a little more investment might have enabled things to work out.

My bike will be travelling with us because I don't have one waiting in Holly's basement. I'll need some way to get around at the other end and jobless will mean carless. It will naturally cost more to put the bike on the plane than I paid for it in the first place but I've got fond of it. I think I'll call it Victoria. Job number two will be working out how to get Vicky to the airport.

Then there's the traditional fret about how we can possibly have collected more junk. And the ever more frequent fume about how hard it is to be itinerant with the sort of luggage one buys when one thinks one is emigrating. The monster suitcase (with wheels) is something of a liability these days, I'd be better off with a backpack.

I need to schedule a couple of last minute banana slug hunts as well and find a way to tell Hinge and Bracket we are leaving. When all that's done I must make time to write to Mum and tell her what we're up to. Poor mother has had an anxious time. Hinge won't answer the phone you see. He won't allow Bracket to answer the phone. There were indeed more house rules and this was the biggest. The kitchen telephone extension must remain unplugged so that the boarders can't hear it ring. All calls go through to the ansaphone in Hinge's room, which only Hinge is allowed to play back. Bracket tells me that he doesn't want her to find out that he's in debt. I am forever getting messages along the lines of 'Joe phoned this morning, could you ring him back before ten because he's going out.' Or 'Can you attend an interview at two-thirty this afternoon?' Hinge checks his messages once a day, at about seven-thirty in the evening. Mother has given up trying. Why waste an international call to tell a machine she rang?

I'm beginning to see why Hinge and Bracket's boarders are few and far between. And why they were so keen to accommodate us so reasonably for an extended period. While I'm on the subject maybe I should offload about mealtimes. No, I'll do that after we have gone, it might be funny by then.

If they let us out. I am also beginning to understand why boarders are so important to the establishment. Hinge and Bracket clearly hate each other with the kind of smouldering resentment that requires a third party to deflect each day's quota of ire on both sides. Without boarders they would most certainly have done away with each other by now. We are the equivalent of those bits of racing car that fly off in a crash; we absorb impact. In fact, I am not at all sure that some of our predecessors aren't stashed away under the floorboards for emotional emergencies.

The one thing I don't need to worry about is the cost of the flight, our air miles bought us a return flight so we may be approaching penniless but we are still travellers.

And when we get there? What then? When we were planning our BC experiment Theresa insisted on us coming back to K/W and staying with them for a while if it didn't work out, so we're going to use our last freebie to take up her offer and be cosseted while I try to summon up the enthusiasm for another burst of jobhunting. I feel in my water (as somebody's auntie used to say) that the adventure is almost over and that we are actually on our way home to England via old friends. Well, new friends that now feel like old ones. But we're beginning to view being homesick for Ontario as the big achievement, no-one can fit in everywhere after all. We're going to leave BC to the beautiful people, I've never been one before and it's a bit late to start now. Leaving Joe will be difficult but that's another chapter.

You pissed me off is seeing us out in style though:

> *-TO THE Swine who stole my coffee cup: I hope you get an incurable disease and that a prized body part turns green and falls off!*

Carolyn Steele

Did I mention that Victorians take their coffee very seriously? Must be something to do with it being so hard to get a proper drink.

* * *

I've had a phone call from Human Resources Canada. They have decided that I am entitled to look for work after all, they would just like to be convinced now that I have been. Please could I send them the yellow form that lists all the jobs I've applied for? Fortunately I'd made a good job of it, every contact religiously recorded. Unfortunately it seems to have disappeared during the packing. I spent my last day in British Columbia at the *Times Colonist* offices, digging out six weeks worth of classified ads from their archives in order to reinvent the jobhunting list. That left me with just about enough time for a fond farewell to the Cheesecake Cafe – my companion chose the Strawberry Daiquiri cheesecake; a classic of its genre and quite sufficient for two – and it was time to buy Joe a book, buy Ben a poster, tell Joe how soon we'd be back, tell Ben how soon we'd be gone and rearrange the bags again.

Rearranging the bags is something of a tradition now. I pack two days before we go anywhere these days, which is quite a progression from two weeks before we left England for the first time last year. Then I rearrange it all the night before, go to bed happy that just the toothbrushes and Bugs Bunny shower gel squeegee will require attention in the morning and repack it all again when I get up. Simple.

Getting Vicky to the airport was a breeze, I'd forgotten how big the cabs are, she popped effortlessly into the boot. Getting her on the plane was another matter entirely. When I telephoned the airline to ask about being accompanied by wheeled transport they told me how much it would cost. They didn't tell me about all the abstruse things you are supposed to do by way of preparation, such as turning handlebars around for flatter packing and letting the air out of the tyres so that they don't pop. All the turning and flattening came as a nice surprise at the check-in desk. The tyres were easy, I did them straight away but the handlebars presented more of a problem. No tools. The combined co-operation of Canadian Regional Air ground staff was mobilised. They rang around the airport and found a bod in the Air Cargo building who had the required set of hex-wrenches. The Air Cargo building was on the other side of the airport. It would have been quicker to cycle there but some idiot had let all the air out of the tyres. We just made the flight in time, all breathless and frazzled and not at all intrepid.

'Didn't you and your son fly to London last year?' asked the stewardess.

'Goodness, do you recognise every passenger?'

'Not usually but I remember taking your little boy to visit the flight deck.' It appears we now have our own cabin staff.

Theresa met us at the airport. The only Crystal Tipps in the arrival hall. Hugs all round and we are back on the bit of roadway outside Pearson Airport where so many people get their first glimpse of Canada. Including the Yank in *Due South*, who couldn't believe seeing two guys on that very bit of kerb arguing over who should offer the other first ride in the only available cab.

Another hallway with our luggage in it. Another spare mattress on the floor. And a lot of mixed feelings. Was it living in BC that got us down or living out of a suitcase? Difficult to tell. A big bit of both of us wants to have a home again; but another big bit wants to see what'll happen next if we don't. Which bit will win is anybody's guess right now, especially since I have received rather mixed news on the money front. My day ferreting around the ex-classifieds paid off to a certain extent, British Columbia Human Resources are now convinced that I'm fully entitled to a spot of cash, backdated to sometime. But we've moved province. I popped into the local jobcentre today to notify them of my change of address. They will request the file from Victoria and review my eligibility.

'But it's just been reviewed' I helpfully pointed out.

'Ontario will have to review it again' the lady insisted.

'What about the back pay they decided I was entitled to?' Guess what? They're going to review it again.

'Why did you move?'

'I ran out of money. I almost had a job. If they'd decided I was entitled to UI a week earlier I could have afforded to stay and wait for it.'

Now I know I'm only a foreigner and all that but this is all starting to feel a little Kafkaesque. It is clearly time to ring every agency in the phone book so they can tell me they can't help. I'm bound to need another list of phone calls to prove I'm really looking for work sometime soon. The real job hunt will take place through Holly and Theresa and their kindness, willingness to help and numerous contacts in the care industry but I have a feeling that won't count.

EIGHTEEN

Another new career

Something turned up. No really. I have accidentally become a chauffeuse. How? Well, Theresa's parents run a limousine company. They had a driver quit on a Friday night, which was extremely inconvenient as regards Saturday's bookings. Panic, followed by brainwave. 'Carolyn used to drive an ambulance. She must be able to handle a limo.' So late in the evening Theresa received an unlikely phone call from her Mum. 'What do you mean you want to speak to Carolyn?' Did I want to drive for fourteen hours the following day? You bet I did. A quick tour round the block to find out how big my new baby was (big), a crash course in etiquette, a rummage through suitcases to find something that could pass for a uniform at a pinch and I was off to sweep a blushing bride to her nuptials in the morning.

There's a lot to remember I'll have you know, apart from where the corners are. There are buttons for divider screens, air conditioning, sunroof and TV. There are buttons to disable the aforementioned gadgets if your client looks as though they will play with things/cause trouble by hanging out of the sunroof/make out and ruin the suspension if they think you can't see them. There's making sure the champagne glasses don't fall over, there's remembering to get the bubbly out of the boot at the right moment. Ditto the pom-poms. There's always walking round the back of car, never the front (your party does not wish to see you shambling about, they wish you to appear at their door as if from nowhere) parking the right way round, never driving into a place you can't manoeuvre out of (in my case, pretty much anywhere) and most important of all, never appear to be lost. Appearance is all, getting lost is inevitable but panache must save the day. There's also enabling a becrinolined bride to shovel herself inside as elegantly as possible, dress, train, big hair and all, remembering not to shut any bits of billowy white stuff in the door. And even more vital than not appearing lost; making sure she doesn't spill her bubbly all down billowy white stuff on the way. Bert explained the technique to me in excruciating detail; Anticipating traffic light changes far enough ahead so that you never need to brake to a complete stop, as few speed changes as possible… 'Don't worry Bert, I'll give her a spinal injury drive, put a glass of champagne on the roof if you like.'

Once this wedding was through I had to go and pick up a bunch of high school kids from a 'prom'. This was a new one on me but I now know that it's a sort of formal dance to celebrate having 'graduated' from school. Although coming from a land where only graduates graduate I am a little bemused by the idea. Leaving school isn't exactly difficult, surely you just get old enough?

One of the main purposes of a prom seems to be to spend as much money as possible on clothing which will only be worn once. The other major point of promming? This would appear to be the undertaking of as much under-age alcohol consumption as possible in one evening. They are not allowed to do this in their limo, there are company rules about it. Unfortunately there is nothing one can do to stop them downing whatever they please outside their limo at each and every party they drop into on the way to and from the event itself.

The issue of whether anyone would vomit before the end of proceedings was one that exercised all our minds a great deal. The kids had a small obsession with the $200 clean-up fee and I was anxious to find out if my vomit-magnet jinx would follow me here. NHS ambulances, private medical standbys, chums at parties, wherever I am the carrots and tomato skin will fly. Without fail. Yours truly holds the record for the fastest sick bag in the UK. And – I'm pleased to report – the fastest ice bucket in North America. My jinx is alive and well and we didn't spill a drop.

During my absence developing the next new career (the accent is proving popular and good for tips) Ben has been entertaining the troops with stories of mealtimes chez Hinge and Bracket. It did get funny quite fast once we no longer had to endure them. Bracket never wanted boarders you see, it was all Hinge's idea but she had to do all the work and he didn't give her enough money to feed us all on. Cue a daily public show of subtle resentment and where better than at the meal table? Hinge and the boarders are presented with a proper 'meat and two veg.' sort of square meal, while Bracket settles down to something cheap and cheerful with many a wistful sigh and sidelong glance. Nothing is said but plenty is implied. Sometimes Bracket's short rations involve a toasted ham and cheese sandwich, more often a bowl of plain pasta. As you picture this scene please bear in mind that Bracket's square meals consist mainly of interesting ideas with cabbage. In addition I think that Hinge is to understand that there is not enough money for seasonings. Ben and I would both have killed for a bowl of plain pasta or a ham and cheese sandwich. Without ham. Or cheese.

Carolyn Steele

There was only ever one spoken reference to the nightly culinary inequity; on the evening in question we were regarding our sausages somewhat dubiously after discovering them to be a bit raw in the middle when Hinge enquired as to their provenance. Bracket prevaricated a little, clearly lost for a way to tell Hinge how cheap they had been and reassure us that they were especially nice at one and the same time. We all agreed in the end that they were a marvellous find of a new line that the local butcher was offering at a trial price. Bracket sighed deeply. 'They *smell* lovely.' They clearly smelt better than they tasted but to this day, neither Ben nor I can look at a sausage on a plate without quietly intoning 'they *smell* lovely.'

In an effort to explain to Ben why some people persist in making each other miserable in subtly ingenious ways I introduced the concept of martyrdom as a personality trait. 'We call it playing the martyr when you want to make someone miserable but you don't want to do anything bad that they can criticise. So you do things to show that they are making you miserable instead. Then they feel bad but can't shout at you. Learn to spot people who do it, then you'll be able to avoid marrying one.' He learned well.

'Mum, you're being a martyr, stop it.'

'Sorry dear.'

* * *

And now to business, because here is the plan. No here's the background to the plan, the plan follows shortly. There are jobs for nannies and live-in carers aplenty and they all think I'm wonderful but no-one has room for an extra small person. It's almost two months since I worked as a carer, which means that any job I do land is unlikely to count towards a whole year of residency (I'll refrain from filling several pages with what does and doesn't make foreigner workers acceptable, suffice it to say I'm an

204

unlikely candidate just now) so we need to decide when to go home. It looks as though I can earn enough haring about in limos to keep us ticking over for a short while so – and here's the plan – we're going to muddle about here for the summer, making the most of the weather and trying to earn enough for one last glorious train ride through the Rockies. Then we'll return to England in time for Ben to start the school year in September. With his old pals. Which might just make it feel a bit better.

In the meantime we're on the move again. Remember Computer Hero? Yes I know I never learn but he needs a childminder. So off we go to do a spot of baby-sitting in lieu of rent. Any comments along the lines of 'a man in every province' will be met with a most severe frown, this time it's strictly business. It will also cheer Ben up. He really fancies the idea of going to school with a kid he knows for a change. After the horrible time he had in Sooke I'm inclined to let him choose our next location. There aren't many weeks of term left, he may as well enjoy them.

I feel sort of duty bound to defend my virtue here, as it occurs to me that I am unlikely to mention this latest move to Joe. I am not noted for my success with the menfolk, clearly an English accent is more exotic than I had imagined. Anyway, for what it's worth, I fell in love properly and stupidly during my last sojourn in K/W and got hurt. It's possible that we hurt each other, that's difficult to guess and I am unlikely to ever be told. However, moving in is a good and sensible idea from the practical point of view. I'd like to think that I am grown-up enough to cope and a bit less vulnerable now I've caught up on sleep and don't require a social life as an aid to sanity preservation. It is entirely possible that I am wrong on both counts, in which case there will be the sort of tears that are better forgotten than written about.

Joe accidentally became, is, and will I suspect always remain, the best friend in the world. It was sad to leave but there was no pain. Given the choice I would clearly prefer to be emotionally tortured than fed and watered. This is patently absurd and in a way I am quite relieved that I will leave them both in the end. In the meantime I will declare notches on the headboard, pretend the next few weeks will be easy and blame the mid-life crisis that dragged us here in the first place.

* * *

It's remarkable how many things can go wrong in a limo. Take this week's wedding for example. Everything was fine until the photographs. It seems to be a tradition here for everyone to swarm to the nearest park or beauty spot for an hour or several to take piccies between the ceremony and the reception, such places as a tree in a churchyard or the steps outside a registry office are not sufficiently picturesque for Canadian wedding albums. Bottles of wine go too and it all takes ages, so when the groom's mother asked me to run her home to collect some desserts and take her – plus desserts – to the reception while the photographer was busy with the big hairs and dresses in the park, it seemed like a good idea. We wouldn't be long after all. I should have smelt a rat when the rest of the groom's family hopped in too. The desserts weren't quite ready you see. An ideal opportunity for the chaps to break open the brandy and cigars. And coffee. And to sample the puds. More coffee? Don't mind if I do.

We weren't quite late yet as it began to rain but the reception was on the other side of town and several scantily clad young ladies were now stranded in the park getting wet until their car returned to rescue them. I finally persuaded sundry coffee and brandy drinkers that we should go or they might miss out on even more booze and we were off. Phew. Then we passed the Canadian equivalent of Woolworth's whereupon the groom's mum yelled 'stop!' I stopped, fearing imminent heart attack or possibly leaky puds. She jumped out of the car and disappeared into the shopping mall. To buy an envelope. Of Greek extraction, she had suddenly decided that an envelope was essential for placing money in to pin to the bride's dress during the dancing. It was a Saturday afternoon, the car park was full and an elderly stretch Chevy has the turning circle of an aircraft carrier. I can now tell you that not only will I place a vomit bag in my pocket before the next prom, I will also secrete an envelope about my person next time a wedding booking bears a Greek surname. I can also tell you that my vehicle's similarity to an aircraft carrier extends to its momentum when loaded and speeding. The desserts almost survived.

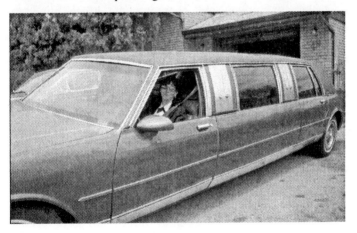

Limousine Sir?

Having a sort of job and a sort of home, give or take a bit of bruised ego, is proving good for us. Ben is back in school. He refused to let me take him on day one, walking along with a pal was too much of a novelty, I sent a note to his teacher explaining that it wasn't that I didn't want to meet her. He brought home a French worksheet with *trez bien* on it. We like this school, he's not had a *trez bien* for anything before.

Life is almost normal again. With the possible exception of grocery shopping on a bicycle. I've rather taken to cycling around K/W. Push-bikes aren't trendy here like they are in Victoria but at least the roads are flat. And very wide. You see more too, I have my favourite gardens on much-cycled routes now. Occasionally one of these will be sporting a gardener as I pootle by. I've taken to appreciating their glorious variegated irises out loud. Most get over their surprise fast enough to offer a weak grin.

The checkout staff at the local supermarket are getting used to their pet mad cyclist too. It takes a little logistical effort to organise the weight distribution you see and they never let you bag your own shopping here. I feel obliged to explain why I'm rearranging their carefully packed carriers, I'd hate for anyone to think me ungrateful but the flat things have to go all together for piling high on the back, then the squishables go separately in bags of equal weight for the handlebars. It's a bit wobbly but pretty foolproof so long as I don't stop all the way home.

And I'm back to scouring *The Record* for snippets of Canadiana to delight and amuse. It's provincial election time in Ontario. I have begun to follow the campaigns with increasing interest now I have realised I don't need a great deal of political background to understand it all. It's just like home. The TV debate between the three main party leaders could so easily have taken place in England. The Tories promised tax cuts, the opposition promised spending on education and health and the no-hoper quibbled. The only difference seems to be that the Tories and Liberals are the main contenders with the left-wingers – the NDP – almost completely marginalised.

The Tories romped home, as expected. The province is remarkably prosperous just now with massive growth and job creation predicted, most people clearly regard cuts in hospital staffing levels and annual teachers' strikes as a price worth paying. Not a cynical comment that, just an observation. If life weren't good here we wouldn't be sad about leaving. The people with most to worry about over the next four years are those receiving welfare benefits. Mike Harris, the returned Premier and foot-in-mouth king, has made no secret of paring welfare to the bone. Remember the pregnant women who might spend their nutrition allowance on beer? His latest scheme is to introduce mandatory drug testing for all welfare recipients.

I know I'm an outsider and have no right to an opinion but this does send a bit of a shiver down my spine. It sounds perilously close to blaming the poor for their poverty and punishing them with a removal of civil liberties. A recent international survey much quoted in the papers here at the time rated Canada as having the highest quality of life in the world. Which is presumably why there aren't enough poor people to have an effect on the ballot box.

And to see an almost-normal week out in style, the next limo fiasco. My windscreen wipers died on the way to the airport this week. In a downpour. At 5.30 in the morning. I was tempted to slow down and try to get there anyway but a bright spark in the back had the temerity to notice and ask if it was safe. My esteemed passengers never normally pay any attention to the sharp end. I tinkered for a while, more for show than anything else, I don't have the foggiest idea how to fix anything more complex than a light bulb. Then I rather shamefacedly put them in a cab and made my own way home very slowly. And I'm pleased I did now, had I been moving at any speed I might have missed a roadside sign that made me laugh out loud. 'Next right. Y2K compliant firewood.' I will never again observe that Canadians have no sense of humour.

NINETEEN

Proper plans

Turtles. I was manoeuvring the limo along an unmade farm track last night in the middle of a spectacular thunder storm when a couple of enormous turtles appeared in the headlights waddling up the road. And what a hypnotising waddle. I couldn't drive around them because of ditches on either side of the track. As I sat mesmerised, one of them helpfully toppled into a ditch but the other continued on his way.

I calculated that at the speed he was travelling he would probably be safe from the rear wheels if I could get him centred between the front ones, I just didn't know what the clearance under the car was. These long stretch efforts bounce around a lot on uneven surfaces but it seemed the only answer so I crawled forward over him (her? it?) waiting for the crunch.

No crunch came, and ten minutes later when I drove back down the lane after delivering my cargo the monster was still ambling happily along the road. I mentioned this to Theresa the following day. She grinned. 'I tried that with a skunk once. I wasn't so lucky, spoiled the wedding a bit.' She also reassured me that any other course of action – getting out and picking it up say, to put it out of harm's way – would have been seriously silly. 'They're Snapping Turtles, you'd have lost a finger or two.' Glad I know that. It had been on my mind as an option, the only reason I didn't was because of the storm.

There are thunderstorms because of the heat wave. And I've learned another few weather phrases. First there is the humidex. This is the hot weather equivalent of the wind chill factor in winter. The weather forecasts give you the temperature first, then tell you how much hotter it will feel because of the humidity. That's the humidex. Currently thirty-six degrees. That's hot. And humid. Hot and humid means thunderstorms, which I now know can be tornadic if hot and cold fronts collide. A tornadic storm doesn't guarantee you a tornado of course, it just means the conditions are right. A baby tornado hit Toronto this week. Strictly speaking it was a twister, a sort of tornadette. Or is that a kind of steak?

There are media warnings for people with breathing or heart problems to stay indoors and a lot of activities are being cancelled, school sports days for example. The risk of dehydration in school time outweighs the benefit of sporting activity in an Ontario summer. Will more things be cancelled due to the heat than the cold? I think it might be close. The population of K/W had taken to shopping in a big way, the malls are almost bustling and the coffee shops are verging on busy. Why? The shopping malls are air-conditioned, it's the only place to while away a superheated afternoon. Usually, when it gets this bad the City Council outdoor staff work shorter hours but not this year. They've been on strike recently – baseball matches have been called off all over the place due to striking groundsmen – and apparently there's such a backlog of work to be done that the City has insisted they continue to work through the heat. I'm not sure this will contribute greatly to harmonious industrial relations but I can imagine the grin on the face of the individual who thought of it.

Clearly the only place to be at such a time is inside an air-conditioned limousine. And I've learned another little routine this week, collecting people from the airport. Far more complicated than you'd think I'll have you know. First you have to find The Compound. This is where all the limos herd together for company and wait to be summoned. It's round the back of Terminal Three, with a nicely hidden entrance so that if you don't know exactly when to turn you're off round the one-way system again. Then you take a slip of paper to the man in the hut – who clearly thinks that women in charge of limousines are causing the breakdown of society as we know it – pay seven bucks, tell him which flight you're meeting and get a reference number. When your bod is through customs – I should really refer to one's party now I'm so experienced – they tannoy your number. All you have to do then is negotiate the turn out of the compound without demonstrating that actually women in charge of limos are causing the breakdown of society as we know it, and find your terminal first time round the one-way system.

The Compound is a good place to see the lesser-spotted limo driver in natural habitat. I'm trying to work out why every chauffeur I've met over here reminds of an ambulance driver I once knew over there. There's the lanky clown who clearly spends his free time leaving his hat out in the rain and then sitting on it, then there's the four-foot-square lady in her fifties with fierce hair, the slightly dim and very spotty youngster who thinks that a uniform makes him look sexy and there's the spiv. Every ambulance station had one of each. And they're all here in the compound at Pearson Airport too. Why? Do the same characters end up driving for a living the world over? And which one am I? Come to think of it, ever since the invention of paramedics, individuals with personalities have disappeared from ambulances to be replaced by energetic clones with buzz cuts. Clearly this is where we have all gone. I'll have to do a bit of chauffeuring when I get home to confirm the theory.

Airport runs are a good opportunity to catch up on *The Archers*. Yes, believe it or not, my mailings of cassettes of the Sunday Omnibus edition are still going strong. There was a bit of a gap during our recent movings around but a huge backlog has just caught up with me. How do you say thank you for such devotion? Linda Snell and her aromatherapy course, Peggy Wooley disapproving of the lady vicar's sponsored walk, Mike Tucker helping Pat through her depression, it's all heavenly. Guess I'm still helplessly English. At least I can look forward to having the Beeb back soon.

Helplessly English despite finally succumbing to syrup. It's taken a long while to get over my inbuilt resistance to Maple Syrup on things I have grown up thinking of as savoury and I still can't quite cope with the idea of splurging it on bacon but I had a go at combining it with French toast the other morning. The ultimate Canadian breakfast, I have taken to making mountains of the stuff for weekend brunches now that I have access to an unmuddy kitchen and people to cook for. The Maple Syrup sat there looking at me and I had to try it. Not bad. Ben, who took against Maple Syrup almost as soon as we got here and hasn't eaten any since, tried it too and declared it good. We have a brand new Canadian family tradition for Sunday breakfast. Just in time to leave the country.

Yes, the plan firms up. We now have a date for starting the convoluted trek home. And a list of things to do for the last time. The limo business will apparently take a nose-dive at the end of June, no more proms after the end of term and too hot for weddings, so this will be time to begin the end.

We'll spend the first part of July revisiting old haunts and packing our belongings into cunningly organised boxes ready for shipping. Then we'll wave good-bye to all but the essentials and jump on a plane. Not home straight away, we have a bit of money left so it has to be back to Vancouver. We can see all the things we missed the first time round due to jet lag. After a week in Vancouver we'll board a train bound for Edmonton, because it's the other side of the Rockies and is where the train stops. Edmonton's only claim to fame is the largest shopping mall in the world. It has an indoor rollercoaster (largest in the world, natch) a beach and four submarines. This is more that the Canadian Navy can muster. Once you've read that don't you absolutely have to see the place? If only to see if it's as nasty as it sounds.

Then we'll fly home. ETA Blighty, first week in August. We will be a few week early as the tenants vacate our house in September but Mum appears to be happy to put us up for the duration. Not a bad plan as it turns out, I will get an interlude of in-house baby-sitter, i.e. serious partying, before the unwelcome business of nest refeathering and English jobhunting. That may soften the blow a bit.

Now we've made the decision, we're sort of looking forward to getting back – having our own home round us, our things, our rules, our mess and our normality – but we're disappointed as well. We wanted to find a way to stay and generate our own normality here one day, stay and learn to blacksmith and lacemake and woodturn. It didn't work and we're very sad. I have a feeling it'll take a lot of parties.

* * *

So I said to Theresa, 'I've got to go to the airport tonight. I hope something goes wrong, I'm running out of things to write about.' She laughed.

215

'Airport runs are too straightforward for trouble.' Then she went away for the weekend. I'll bend her ear when she returns.

It all started with the car making a funny noise. As soon as I switched it on fortunately, rather than half way along Highway 401. We dithered and deliberated and decided it shouldn't really go to Toronto while it was bleeping. Frantic phone calls to all the other local limo companies produced one available car but no-one to drive it. 'That's OK, I've got a driver, she's on her way to collect it.'

I was supposed to pick up a family in Waterloo at 10.30, run them to the airport in time to meet their Grandma off her plane at 11.45 and bring everybody home again. By the time I eased myself into the replacement vehicle 10.30 had been and gone. Now this is going to sound really girly and stupid but it turned out to be a Lincoln and so far I'd only driven Chevys. The buttons are in different places. I found all the woofers and tweeters in the end but it took a good while. I rushed to collect my people. They wouldn't have been far away if someone hadn't demolished the Ottawa Street bridge over the Expressway while I wasn't looking. It was definitely there when we left town a few months ago. Irritable family finally collected at 11.15. With many a reassurance about how long it takes to get through customs and collect one's luggage I soothed their fears about Grandma being kept waiting and loaded them into the car.

That's when the awful truth dawned. There was one bit of apparatus I hadn't found. The wossname for switching power on in the back. No lights, air conditioning, radio, TV, in fact no toys for my passengers to play with at all. Family beyond irritable, verging on irate. 'Not my usual car' I muttered, 'must have been disconnected for proms, can't trust kids not to break stuff...I'll see to it when we get there...no time now...lets get you to meet Grandma.' and off we sped. We only saw the speed limit once on the way and that was while passing a police car. I got them there at five past midnight. Not bad, just time enough to pop round to the compound, act pathetic and persuade another driver to help me find the errant thingumy while Gran finishes clearing customs. All planes are late aren't they? Grandma would have her toys on the way home and all would be well. I might even get a tip.

So what are the odds on any particular plane arriving a whole hour early? I'd really like to know. Ours never do. Grandma had been waiting a very long time. No nipping to the compound for advice, so back we went sans toys. No tip. The only cheering thought during the entire nightmare was that owner of my replacement car had said he might need a driver sometime, I should leave him my phone number when I returned the car. In the interests of earning as much as I can before we leave so we can afford our last spot of sightseeing I decided to do this. I locked my number and the keys inside the car as instructed. Then I realised I'd left his lights on. Guess he won't be employing me after all. I did find out how to switch power to the back though, accidentally, as I parked up at the end of the night. Not a wossname or a thingumy after all, you flip the ignition switch. Glad I know that.

* * *

School's out. Yes, the great Canadian summer holiday has begun and parents are asking each other if they think they'll cope. No more school means no more proms, everyone has 'graduated' now and presumably the lesser-spotted limo driver will be in more limited demand. I shall declare myself on holiday and book flights, trains and motel rooms.

If I can be bothered. It's hot. The humidex is terrifying. Even my hair is sweating.

TWENTY

The beginning of the end

It's Canada Day. Again. The dear place is 132 years old and the nation will wish it happy birthday every way it can: military fly-pasts in Ottawa, huge picnics in Victoria and fireworks up the road after a day of outdoor frolicking. We were too jet lagged to appreciate the enormity last year, waking up in time for the fireworks was as far as we got, so plans were afoot to make the most of this, our second (and last) Canada Day. We would know not to take the car. We would feel like old hands.

Then it rained. A lot. The rain mightn't have put paid to the fireworks on its own but the lightning certainly did. The local radio carried hourly updates on whether the fireworks were likely to go ahead but with the issue still unsettled at seven in the evening we opted to go out for supper instead. The radio assured us that a rain date was fixed for Sunday but in the end the fireworks were put back in their boxes for next year. Apparently it has to be Canada Day or there's no point. Bereft of fireworks there was nothing for it but to go out for supper again. Knocked a couple of 'must try that place before we go's off the list of farewell visits. The *Noodle Factory* was a bit of a let down but *Moose Winooski's* was splendid fun, we might have to schedule a farewell visit now we've found it.

After the thunderstorms, more heat wave. Strange weather, nay big weather, is in the news again. We've got it easy here really, it's just too hot to move, the hospitals are filling up with heat related collapses and I am typing very slowly in order to minimise the sweating. Elsewhere in Ontario life is more exciting, at one and the same time a house was struck by lightning in Cambridge and a tornado spread trees and barns across the countryside near Duncan.

Alberta is breaking records too. There were sixty centimetres of summertime snow between Jasper and Banff in the mountains while snow-melt flooding swamped the foothills. The Prairies are flooded too – torrential rain there as opposed to snowmelt – and it's pretty wet in British Columbia. That's not unusual though, it's always pretty wet in British Columbia.

The newspaper carried a handy article on lightning strikes this week after a lady golfer was struck in Edmonton. Did you know that about twelve Canadians a year die from being struck by lightning? And that you can be hit as far as thirty-five kilometres away from a thundercloud? That's why you're supposed to stay indoors for half an hour after the storm has passed. While staying indoors you should avoid dealing with water or wiring. No showers, washing up or tinkering with the TV cable. So Auntie Win was right all those years ago to unplug the telly in a storm. You shouldn't even use the phone for goodness sake, why didn't I know all this before? I've been risking life and limb by ringing Theresa for a chat within half an hour of a thunderstorm. I might be sad to leave but it'll be quite comforting to get back to non-life-threatening weather.

And the preparing to leave continues, Ben is getting himself psyched up for home by taking cooking lessons. His passion for French toast (with syrup) has extended to learning to make the stuff. I am pleased. Not only because boys should be able to feed themselves or because he's taken to cooking my breakfast but mainly because he's practising for showing his English friends what Canadians like to eat. It's good to see him putting a positive spin on going home.

We're beginning to think souvenirs as well. What should we make sure to have for ever to remind us we once nearly lived here? Which bits of Canada ought we to take home? What will still mean something once we have settled down and half forgotten most of it? (Apart from the totally practical extreme weather gear we've collected along the way, I'll probably get more long-term satisfaction from my nineteen dollar fleecy-lined leather bootees than anything else if I'm honest but they seem a bit prosaic just now.) Nothing that says 'I've been to Canada' on it for a start, that would be thoroughly unBritish and we will have to relearn being sophisticated, reserved and unfriendly very soon. The souvenir question is much more emotionally demanding than such trivia has a right to be. It involves thinking about being back in the old routine. It is shelved for a while.

We really are doing things for the last time now, in between packing boxes. One day a poignant revisit to Blue Mountain, the next an educational interview with the freight company about bicycles. It would appear that putting Vicky on a boat is more complicated than putting her on a plane. It's not just turning the handlebars this time, it's taking the pedals off. In a spirit of total defeatism I rang the local bike shop and was delighted to discover that for the vast sum of twenty bucks they'll dismantle, pack and deliver both bikes by next Tuesday. For once I think I'll do something the easy way.

That will free up some time to make a packing list the hard way. Yes the educational freight company have mentioned Customs. Apparently the inventory I left in Holly's basement (was it only a couple of months ago?) isn't detailed enough, I'll have to open all the boxes and start again. And have an internal tussle over the Cinnamon Schnapps. Remember the Cinnamon Schnapps? I discovered on Christmas Eve that is isn't actually very nice. No wonder Santa left most of his. There's about three-quarters of a bottle left and it would hardly be worth packing except that it's a Christmas present, a gift from Ally and therefore of sentimental value. And there are all these little gold flakes in the bottom of the bottle. Naturally Ben has his eye on these. The sensible solution would be to pour the contents away and save the flakes but I have an inbuilt resistance to wasting booze, even when it's nasty. In the box it went in the end, I've paid for the minimum square metreage so I may as well fill it up. I dutifully added 'part of an opened bottle of spirits' to the inventory.

The sunset was spectacular the day we said good-bye to Blue Mountain. The sunset was spectacular the day we said good-bye to Niagara Falls too and Toronto, I've spent a lot of time saying 'I'll miss the sky'. And eating sweet corn. We won't be able to buy corn cobs fresh from the farm gate by the dozen much longer and it's such wonderful stuff. Totally different to the tough old things we knew at home. 'And why is that?' I hear you ask. I'll tell you why, these amazing cobs are genetically modified that's why. Three minutes in boiling water, no need for salt or butter, genetically modified to be scrumptious beyond belief.

Not very politically correct I grant you but that's a non-debate in Canada. People are mildly surprised that the UK thinks it's a bad thing, why pay more for organic when you can pay less for GM? I can see their point. I think I'm going to miss proper corn back home as much as I've missed decent cheese over here. Oh well, there's a consolation. What'll I start with? Applewood smoked, Red Leicester, Sage Derby?

The farewell visit to Toronto produced a new little delight. As well as all the usual stuff – going ooh and ahh up the CN Tower and playing on the streetcars – we set off into one of the less salubrious parts of town in search of a street corner where people play chess. We found it eventually, tucked away behind a row of shops full of ethnic clothing and toe rings. Out on the sidewalk there's a clutch of concrete tables and seats. You'd be forgiven for thinking it was a picnic area, until you spot that the tables are square, there's only one seat each side and on the top, a tiled mosaic marks out a chess board. It takes a while to take all this in because of the crowds. Each table has a game in progress and a rapt audience.

You get the feeling that a lot of the 'chess fans' would be hanging around on the opposite corner sniffing the contents of crisp packets if there wasn't any chess to watch but I found that rather encouraging. Given that guys will be guys and hang around on street corners anyway, they may as well do something constructive. Ben was fascinated by the timed game. Each player had a little stop clock that had to be smacked with much gusto as he made his move. Eventually one of the players stood aside so that Ben could have a game. I thanked him for his kindness. And I thanked the other chap for his patience in being prepared to waste his time playing a child.

You'll have to forgive me if I engage doting mother mode here for a sentence or two because Ben actually won his game, earning a ripple of applause from a street corner full of unsavoury-looking strangers. Of all the unexpectedly odd things we've got up to I have a feeling that one will stand out for a long time as the oddest. Yet another product of the big geography lesson, not only can he protect himself from seismic aftershocks, he can challenge crusty strangers with alcoholic noses to games of chess on street corners and win. This will no doubt come in handy for Key Stage Two.

* * *

My new improved slimline packing routine has gone to pot. I've spent hours camped out in Holly's basement packing and repacking, arranging and rearranging, scribbling changes to the customs list and getting fretful. The train journey complicates things you see. On the one hand I've paid to send bulk the equivalent of a sizeable fridge home by container so I may as well get my money's worth and send as much as possible. On the other, I don't know what the weather will be like in Vancouver. Or Edmonton. Or London. Maybe I should hang on to some colder weather gear, even a normal summer could feel chilly after the Ontario heat. On the third hand – no I don't have three but you know what I mean – we're not just flying from one city to another and hopping into a cab, anything I don't freight home I'll have to carry on and off The Train and presumably supervise during twenty-three hours of spectacular scenery.

Worrisome questions include: will we want to swim? Can I bear to be surgically removed from the computer? And what has happened to all the socks? There were socks aplenty when we arrived back in Kitchener. I remember packing them. Several times. Admittedly neither of us has worn one, or even two, all summer but that's no reason for them all to have toddled off in disgust. I've had to schedule an emergency sock-shopping trip. Which put me in mind of trainers. They're cheaper here so I detailed Ben to try his old ones on for size. He is of the opinion that they're plenty big enough. Trainers off the list then. I might buy some coffee mugs though. They'd make nicely prosaic souvenirs, a sensibly functional way to remember the fave hangouts. Some from *Harvey's* and some from *Chapters*. Maybe in years to come I'll have a wistful flashback every time I pour a coffee. As opposed to the wistful flashforwards I'm getting now when I do things like wave off the luggage. Watching the boxes go was an odd sensation. I was working up to an attack of pensiveness (pensivity?) when the chap who collected it all dropped the box with my computer in it. I decided instantly to go for the optional extra insurance and to refuse his offer of marriage. Several chaps have suggested this as an option for staying on ('you wouldn't have to live with me or anything') but it sort of feels like cheating.

I seem to remember – a lifetime ago – posing the question 'so what would you do with your last night at home?' Here's the next in the series: what would you do with your last day somewhere you'd learned to love? The single suitcase we had left was packed early, the plane didn't leave until suppertime, so we had a day to fill up with mooching about and trying not to be sad. We ended up in *Chapters* drinking coffee, reading up on Vancouver and making lists of places to visit. Did you know Vancouver has the only classical Chinese garden outside China? It's on the list, along with Stanley Park, Grouse Mountain and an international Fireworkfest that happens to start this week. We plan to spend some time playing on the Skytrain too. Wonder if it'll have signs that say 'Mind the Gap' like the subway does in Toronto. For some reason I always find this extremely funny.

The old excitement of being off to somewhere new had taken hold by the time we hit Pearson airport for the last time, a tad early in order to conduct our patented 'moving from one climate to another' routine. This nifty wheeze involves a carrier bag of jeans, trainers and jumpers and a swift visit to the airport toilet once the air conditioning has cooled us down. Shorts and sandals being lighter to carry and easy to stuff into a handbag, we re-emerge from our

Carolyn Steele

quick change a piece of hand luggage less but not as sweaty and hot as if we'd been in the stuff all day. Clever eh?

Ben reappeared from his transformation saying 'Mum, my trainers are too small.' Oh well, at least we now have something to buy in the world's largest shopping mall. Must remember to ask for running shoes though. Trainers don't exist here, people think you want some bizarre kind of nappy.

TWENTY-ONE

The scenic route home

Ben chatted up a school principal on the plane to Vancouver. I don't know quite how he does it but he returned from an expedition to the toilet with a fan in tow. Egged on by much questioning he spent the remainder of the flight regaling her, her travelling companion and most of the rest of the plane with bits of our life story and snippets of Hinge and Bracket's domestic habits, complete with relatively effective mimes of smouldering resentment. His latest conquest was sufficiently taken with us to insist on driving us from the airport to our motel. She took my phone number as well, in case any parents at her school need a nanny. Yup, pack a kid.

We're back in Beautiful British Columbia and Vancouver is predictably spectacular. The beaches are clean, the buildings are eye-catching, the transit system is efficient and the mountains make every walk a novelty. Not just when you've made an expedition somewhere photogenic, they're round every corner and at the end of every street. You catch mountains out of the corner of your eye as you get off the bus or emerge from the supermarket. I wonder how long it takes before you take them for granted. No-one else seems to walk around with their mouth open.

We had fun on the Skytrain (no gap) it reminded me of the docklands light railway in a lot of ways, apart from the mountains. Had fun on the trolleybuses too, they reminded me of being a very small child and seeing the overhead wires taken down in our part of London, apart from the mountains. We had fun in Stanley Park, especially once we found the free trolley ride, I've hiked through yer actual genuine rainforest once and I felt no compulsion to prove I could do it again. And this one may be in downtown Vancouver but there's still 1,000 acres of it and that's a long walk. Tea-rooms notwithstanding.

I began to realise that we were 'doing' Vancouver because it was on the list. Along with boxing up the bike and remembering to give my mobile phone to Holly. It was a thing-to-do-before-we-went. We weren't rummaging around the town in order to learn how to live there but we weren't quite on holiday either. We were an odd and slightly disgruntled sort of tourist. We weren't to know before we arrived but having already rejected and been rejected by British Columbia was to colour our week.

We admired the Lions Gate Bridge (famous landmark) got the cable car up Grouse Mountain (super view) moseyed around the markets on Granville Island (very trendy) had a guided tour of the Classical Chinese Garden (how can someone possibly speak that slowly?) and had our photos taken by the steam clock in Gastown. An American couldn't have done Vancouver more correctly.

Gastown by the way, according to my guidebook, is named after a somewhat boastful saloon owner known as 'Gassy Jack'. According to the locals it's called Gastown because it was the first part of town to be powered by gas. Disappointing but equally likely eh? Fortunately the steam clock is all it's cracked up to be, i.e. powered by steam. And a very hot and sticky place to stand and have a piccie taken on a warm day. Being steamy and all that, especially on the back of the legs.

Then there's the orientality back again. Signs outside the Chinese restaurants are in Chinese. Just Chinese. No westernised versions of oriental cuisine to attract custom here. I'd been a little sniffy about the Chinese restaurants in K/W because they seemed to serve the sort of MSG-laden goo that English eaters rejected several years ago in favour of dishes we thought were more authentic, so we felt duty-bound to sample a 'really traditional' dim sum while we were here. Never again. Gooey, squidgy, sticky, worryingly unrecognisable and uniformly nasty. We were doing OK until the curried whole baby squid (with tentacles). Ben won my unreserved admiration for trying one, after he'd fought it with chopsticks for a while. I've been completely cured of my superior attitude to 'authentic' food. I like spring rolls and sweet and sour pork actually. Another bit of pompousness punctured. Unlike the squid.

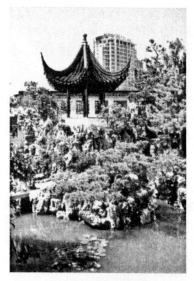

China in Vancouver

Clearly we are back in British Columbia booze-wise. Here's an excerpt from this week's edition of a friendly little publication called *The Buzzer*, published by Vancouver's Transit company for the edification of passengers.

> *Getting to the Fireworks.*
> *Note that the consumption of liquor in public places (including transit vehicles, stations, park & ride lots, public streets and beaches) is illegal. Local police forces will be assisting Translink Special Provincial Constables and other operating staff in monitoring transit vehicles and facilities. Liquor carried on the transit system, whether open or not, is subject to seizure by Transit Constables or local police, in accordance with the BC Liquor Act.*

Must remember to walk back from the shops.

The dry fireworks were popular though. The *Benson and Hedges Symphony of Fire* (odd to be at an event sponsored by tobacco and not allowed to drink, would it be reversed in the UK?) showcases a different three countries each year, all competing to produce the best show, with a joint effort by way of finale. We were around for Canada's display, the first of the series, but had moved on before France and Spain each had their evening of glory so I can't tell you who was best. The fireworks were set up on a big barge thingy in the sea off English Bay beach. Most of Vancouver – 30,000 people according to the *Sunday Province* hopped on buses, trolleys and Skytrains to stake out a little place on the beach, have a picnic maybe, watch the sun go down over the mountains and enjoy the fizz-bangs, set off to the music of a thousand transistor radios playing a simultaneous accompaniment. It was lovely. Just like Alexandra Palace on November the fifth. Except for the mountains of course and the sea and the beach and the sunset and the warmth. And the absence of beer. It took just as long to get home though, what with all the road closures, bottlenecks and overstuffed buses. I'd rather be stuck at a bus stop for hours on a balmy Vancouver evening than in London in November of course but a drinkypoo would have been nice.

Then all of a sudden it was time to revisit the Canadian Pacific Railway Terminus – still love that ceiling – and jump on *The Canadian* because we were finally going to see The Rockies. Ben was most excited to discover the name of the train. Last year his school in Kitchener invited an author called Eric Wilson to talk to the children. Before the visit they'd all read a book of his called *Murder on The Canadian.* And now here we were on the very same train, although hoping to make it without massacre obviously. I was most excited to discover that you could check baggage. I could have brought the computer after all. I then fell to wondering how it was. When I complained to the freight company about the droppage they said 'oh it'll all be dropped a few more times before you see it again.' I'm having to make hand-written notes for goodness sake, on a train, I'll have to get them made up at the chemist.

I'm not a train fanatic. I quite like railway journeys but that's an occupational hazard of generally doing all the driving. So when I say that *The Canadian* is truly stupendous, I do so entirely without the aid of an anorak. It's enormous. I should have counted the carriages shouldn't I? Or befriended a proper enthusiast to tell me how long it is in metres or feet. Saying that it took forever to walk far enough to get to the economy seats just doesn't do it. Sorry.

In addition to being unquantifiably big it has observation cars, glass bubbles up little flights of stairs, perfect for a good view of sunsety and mountainy events as they unfold. The trip is thoughtfully timed to be most viewsome during daylight, leaving at seven in the evening and rattling through the Frazer Valley all evening and most of the night. The big stuff begins shortly after sunrise and continues pretty much all the next day, so we planned to set up camp in the only observation car available for the cheap seats early in the morning.

Once settled back in my numbered seat I was allowed to consume an alcoholic beverage. A lady comes round to take orders occasionally but you have to promise faithfully to stay put until you've finished it and not wander about wantonly waving alcohol and frightening the children. Presumably your seat counts as a putative private dwelling. I ordered a beer, more because I could than because I wanted one and fell to wondering if saving money by sleeping in our seats rather booking a berth was going to prove a false economy. It seemed like it as we tried to get comfortably settled to sleep but oddly enough it turned into a Good Thing the following morning. Sufficiently uncomfortable for me to rise with the dawn (most uncharacteristic) and beat the rush for the bubble while Ben took advantage of my seat to stretch out for an extra hour or so.

And again I'm overwhelmed with the size of this unbelievable country. We crossed a time zone for goodness sake. And the mountains went on. And on. For hours. And hours. I had much clever photography planned but mostly I just sat and gawped. I have run out of suitable adjectives and feel very small.

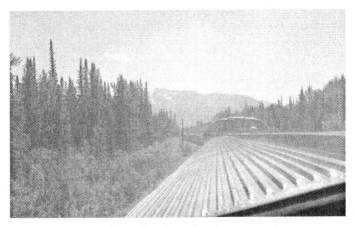

The Canadian from the cheap seats

We arrived in Edmonton at about seven thirty on Monday evening. It was closed.

I asked the cab driver why I could see trolley bus wires but no buses. 'There aren't any really' he said. Then he thought for a while and added 'there'll probably be a few around tomorrow morning.'

I was interested to note that our hotel boasted a bar downstairs.

'Is it OK to take a beer up to my room?' I asked the receptionist.

'They do off-sales' she replied. I thanked her and toddled off to unpack none the wiser. I had in my head the image of a British type of pub-with-off-licence-attached, so when a little thirst took hold I went to explore the building.

The downstairs bar seemed to be all there was so I gave up my search for an off-licence, bought a bottle of *Canadian* and a can of Coke and rejoined Ben, whose job had been to find the cable channel that tells you what's on while I was gone. Well, it was a hot night and we'd been travelling forever, so what with one thing and another it didn't take long before I was ready for another.

'What are you doing with this beer?' demanded the barman. 'Are you taking it to your room?' I was distraught. Had I inadvertently broken some obscure liquor law particular to Alberta?

'I'm sorry, I didn't know, aren't I allowed to?' The barman developed that look on his face that men get when they know you're going to cry in a minute and that it's all their fault but they don't know why.

'It's OK' he said reassuringly, 'if you'd told me, I'd have made it an off-sale, that's all.' There was nothing for it but to come clean.

'You'll have to explain' I confessed, 'I'm a daft Brit fresh from British Columbia where you can't drink anywhere, I've never been to Alberta before and I don't know what you're talking about.' Everyone else in the bar put down their drinks, silenced their conversations and grinned.

It turns out that in Alberta you call it an off-sale if you are removing your chosen beverage from licensed premises unopened. They have to put it in a brown paper bag. Then they charge you A Lot Less for it. The poor chap had wanted to save me a dollar a bottle, not report me to the liquor police. I have a mission now. Some day I have to visit all the provinces we haven't been to yet and find out how to buy a bottle of *Canadian*. (Which, if you are planning a visit by the way, is the only bottle of anything purporting to be lager that tastes of anything other than water. Trust me.)

We found a bus in the morning, although the cabbie was right, there weren't many. And we've now seen West Edmonton Mall. Not only is it the biggest shopping mall in the world (according to the Guinness Book of Records) it also boasts the world's largest indoor amusement park, with the largest indoor rollercoaster (rated #1 in the world for G-force according to the leaflet) the world's largest indoor wave pool, a beach, a lagoon full of fishy exhibits (and Klinger the Giant Octopus) the famous submarines, a casino, several nightclubs and a hotel. Yes, you can holiday there. But would you want to?

Ben had been looking forward to the biggest indoor rollercoaster in the world so we made it our first destination.

'Sheeesh kebab!'

'At least.'

It looped the loop. Three times. I know it's a long way to go to not try the biggest indoor rollercoaster in the world but in our defence, we did watch it for a good while. We submarined past some rather mangy fish tanks and bought some trainers (sorry, running shoes). Then we'd both had enough. It would have been a disappointing day if we hadn't happened by a tiny fossil shop on our way back to the hotel. A shop which, incidentally, ought to be in the Guinness Book of Records for the world's most informative owner. There's a kind of giant Ammonite that's only found in Alberta, which develops incredibly phosphorescent shiny colours as it fossilises. They use it for jewellery. People travel from all over the world to see it. I'm so glad Alberta is famous for something other than a shopping mall.

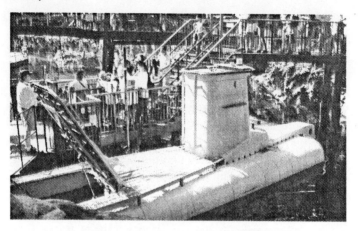

OK, so it's quite a small submarine

TWENTY-TWO

Too loud man

A day in Edmonton before flying home turned out to be a stroke of genius. We didn't mind leaving. It felt more like going home from holiday than abandoning a new and (oddly enough given all the hiccups) much loved country, probably for ever. I was sufficiently untearful on the way to the airport to notice that the dual carriageway sported bales of hay down the middle as well as on both sides. Only in Canada would they make central reservations big enough to farm.

It was a short hop to Calgary and a conveniently quick connection. We just had time to spot the line of chairs we'd snoozed on last time round, then we were Really Leaving. And too tired to give it much thought. We made a half-hearted effort to chat about the people we were looking forward to seeing again, the stories we'd tell, the things it would be fun to unpack, then we stopped bothering and watched the movie. This is unprecedented. Not only are we usually too excited to watch the movie, we usually call it a film. Being eccentrically English for kicks isn't working for us any more.

Then it was over. Just like that. You step off a plane and something is finished. How can that be?

And the noise starts. London is still loud. It was noisy last time we popped home but that was a holiday. This is real life (back to normal?) and that makes it louder. I have a kind of auditory claustrophobia. The houses are too close together and so are the people and everything echoes. I get little panic attacks when people speak. I can see their lips move but I can't hear what they say for the noise of them speaking. And what's more the bus driver doesn't want to know how I am. I'd like everyone to go away and leave me alone. Quietly please.

I know that the cast list of our previous life have missed out on the pleasure of our company – and very awful it must have been for them – but now is not a good time to expect us to entertain. We've got thinking to do. We're not sure if we're still the same people any more, what we need is time to work on it. What we've got is put back into the same pigeonholes. Again.

Curmudgeonly is the word. It's not jet lag – that would be a craven apology of an excuse – it's old fashioned bad temper, the sort that offends people. The best solution seems to be a little self-induced isolation. If we don't see anyone we can't upset anyone. Don't go anywhere, put off the parties, leave the phone to ring. It's bound to be a phase, we'll get bored sooner or later but at least we won't accidentally reject kind words and expressions of welcome and then have to apologise and feel even worse. In fact, being incommunicado for a while will give me time to shout at the shipping agents.

Yes, I have found a suitable target for temper because carting one's belongings round the world isn't as foolproof as it's cracked up to be. I explained carefully to the agent in Kitchener that our boxes were destined for one address but that I would be staying at another. I wrote it down and everything. Twice. I may as well not have bothered because they didn't quite get round to mentioning it to the agent this end. When I dropped into the house one day to see how the lodgers were getting on with moving out so we could move in, I found a letter telling me my beloved Things had been sitting in a warehouse in Tilbury for over a week and I would be liable for storage costs. After seven days.

I rang and cumudgeoned, they apologised. I said I'd drive down there the following day and they said I couldn't. It would take at least three days for the consignment to clear Customs after I'd returned the declaration form they'd enclosed in the letter I hadn't had for a week. The best they could do, they said, would be to generously waive the storage charges if I sent the form back by return and then let me know as soon as Customs were happy. Things would happen quickest, they said, if my packing list was detailed (phew). Then when the officer in charge of checking Ben's Lego for drugs opened a box and found it to be accurately described in excruciating detail he might not bother with the rest. 'It's as good as in the post,' I assured them, picking up my pen and putting down the phone.

Then I read the form. It wanted to know about any alcohol, tobacco or perfume in intimate detail. In other words it wanted to know about my Cinnamon Schnapps. It wanted to know who had distilled it, what percentage proof it was and what size the bottle was for goodness sake. Also an estimation of how much was left (a darned sight too much in my view). I was suffering, by this stage, from excruciating computer separation anxiety. If I didn't supply the relevant information, springing my Things could take weeks the man had said. Presumably therefore, if I omitted to confess to three-quarters of a bottle of glittery gloop, I'd never see the beloved souvenir of my tragically doomed and reason-for-writing-book transatlantic love affair ever again.

I can now report that there isn't an offy in North London that sells Cinnamon Schnapps. I've visited every single one on a hunt for the same bottle so that I could copy the details from a label.

And guess what. I am beginning to regret packing it. No that's a too-English understatement, I'm completely and utterly pissed off with the rotten stuff. Why the hell didn't I pour it carefully through a tea strainer and down an Ontario drain when I had the chance? I know with an awful certainty that I am fated to carry this part-bottle of nastiness wherever I go throughout the rest of my life…I will never drink it and I will never now tip it away because that would make this week's crisis even more pointless.

I finally traced the shop it came from through a ticklish conversation with Ally and rang them up. Try, if you will, to formulate the necessary questions without sounding several burgers short of a barbeque. They didn't laugh or anything, they just dealt with my request very quickly and quietly, as though they were terrified that this odd woman might just *come into the shop* if thwarted.

* * *

The customs form is finally in the post. It'll be next week at the earliest before I see my beloved computer again (oh I do hope it's OK). In the meantime I have a lot of cleaning to do. Yes we're finally home, after seventeen months, seven moves and three schools.

The very last move, from The Mumster's tender care back into our old house, is turning out to be a bit traumatic. Life with Mum wasn't easy, no I'll rephrase that, life for Mum wasn't easy. We were in no way suitable candidates to be lovingly fed and watered by someone who had missed us a lot. Pulling up the drawbridge may have stopped me from offending most people and I guess Mum understands because, well, it's in the job description (although I think a bunch of flowers may be in order) but we really needed to have our home around us for the right kind of cathartic sulk. Or so it seemed. I thought it would all be OK then.

It isn't of course. Things aren't as I left them. How dare things be different? I have a new object of rage and the sort of overwhelming need to scrub the place from top to bottom that one usually associates with chucking out a partner.

'Someone's rearranged the curtains…I left the cupboard under the stairs tidier than this…who moved the rubbish bin?' I know why I'm so angry of course and I know I'm being daft but it's my end-of-adventure and I'll be unreasonable if I want to.

Amid the cleaning binge and associated fury I had an interesting email from Joe. He thought I might be amused. During the second *Benson and Hedges Symphony of Fire* in Vancouver, the authorities set up a checkpoint at the main transit station that serves Downtown and searched everyone. They confiscated all liquor (open or closed) that they found on or about all persons passing through the station. And presumably had a party. Can you imagine that happening anywhere in England without a riot? Can you imagine anyone even suggesting it? It was the first good belly laugh I'd had since getting back and I am eternally grateful to Joe, not only for guessing that I might need a giggle but for knowing me well enough to be sure this would do it. Old pals might still be talking to the wrong person, some doppelganger for whoever I've turned into but if the new friends are real and the changes are real, well maybe it isn't quite all over in the blinking of an eye. In the step off a plane. Just maybe we don't have to climb back into out old pigeonholes if we don't want to.

The boxes, my beloved Things arrived just in time to nurture that little glimmer of hope. And such a spiffy-clean house to unload them into, Christmas in September. The precious computer was unscathed and we'd quite lost track of how many exciting things we'd squirreled away to bring home. We had remembered the obvious stuff, the telescope, the bikes, the industrial quantities of Lego – all those small stashes left in various parts of the world are finally reunited and gosh it's a whole lot of Lego, almost a floorful – and the coffee mugs of course. The real glee came from the things we'd forgotten about.

Ben's special chess set I'd bought him in a fit of parental pride and then not let him use because it was nice. The candleholders we acquired during a very strange day with the Hamilton chapter of the *Society for Creative Anachronism*. The pieces of jade Ben picked up on Vancouver Island, a photo I fell in love with in a tiny art gallery in Tobermory.

My special bargain fleecy boots and silly winter hats. Ben's poster of Victoria that the lady in the launderette gave him because she liked his accent. My copy of *Canajun Eh?* a present from Theresa to help me master the language. In particular to stop her having to wince every time I said Toronto. Phonetically *Tronna*, I still can't do it.

Our souvenirs were working. And, coffee mugs aside, they were not things we bought at the last minute, they were things we had acquired along the wayside. A story in every box. Unpacking was almost like having the good bits all over again and we are nearly happy. There is evidence that we went away, did things and saw stuff. Real physical proof that we have the right to have changed a bit. The tantrums are dying down and we are beginning to be what people expect, full of stories and pictures and tall tales and excellent mimes of smouldering resentment.

Everyone we know now thinks sausages *smell* lovely and poached eggs are a huge joke throughout much of North London, Williegate is now an international phenomenon. The snapping turtles get a little larger with each retelling and bottles of mineral water will forever be earthquake supplies.

I'm getting used to being luv in the shops, instead of ma'am, Ben is preparing a presentation for when he gets back to school – fossils I found all by myself near Lake Huron – and the house has bits of Canada all over it. Including a 'map wall'. We look at it a lot and I have stopped cursing at Ontario maps, they make great wallpaper.

I have my old job back. Yes, I know I didn't want to be put back into old pigeonholes but this is me climbing in voluntarily and I reserve the right to remain irrational a little longer. I'm grateful to the chaps who kept it open for me, they didn't have to and it's a big worry out of the way. One of the things I'd given no thought to at all when swanning off to seek my fortune was how I'd support us when we came home. Income of some sort will be required, I seem to have run up a credit card bill of transatlantic proportions and I've no particular wish to amble into a temp. agency and try to persuade total strangers wearing too much make-up that I may have no measurable typing speed but am a terribly interesting person, would make a fascinating addition to any workplace and have a lot of good stories about sausages and eggs. The old job will do nicely and I'll refrain from moaning about pigeonholes for a while…I have to buckle down and get some thinking done.

It is just possible you see, that this is the beginning and not the end. Going back legally and forever isn't as outlandish a proposition as I had supposed. I've nosed through the leaflets and booklets and bumph and chatted to an immigration consultant and it's sort of feasible. Not easy but not quite out of the question. I can't go and get a job because I'm Not The Right Sort of Person *but*, and this is a much bigger and more significant *but* than I had previously realised, I can go and create employment if I like. Canada wants entrepreneurs. I've looked it up in the dictionary. Now

I know what one is I'm sure I could be one if I put my mind to it. All I need is a lump of capital and a big idea. It would have to be a very big, clever and convincing idea to get past immigration but that's what the consultants are for.

We have had a family conference and decided to give ourselves a year to try and settle down. We will try hard, we will mean it. After all, everyone goes through a phase of wanting to live somewhere else when they come back from holiday don't they? It doesn't normally take long to realise that you wouldn't really like to live in Majorca or Mexico or wherever. Just now we're feeling deprived of so much; clean air, empty roads, safe playgrounds, dead groundhogs, all-you-can-eat garlic bread, City-sponsored ice rinks, the list is endless. Sage Derby cheese and Have I Got News For You just aren't helping at all. But who knows? In a year we are very likely be content again, happily back in our boxes, if a little smugger than before and unaccountably amused by sausages and poached eggs. If so, I'll store up the photographs to inflict on great-grandchildren and try to stop bringing Canada into every conceivable conversation on the flimsiest of pretexts.

If we're still restless, if we still yearn for the air and the space, the skunks and groundhogs, people who say 'howareya?' and 'you're welcome', if Canada is still calling us this time next year, well, then I'll get the house valued and go looking for that big idea. Deciding when to make a decision always feels so decisive doesn't it?

In the meantime we can tell ourselves it needn't be over. I might yet get to be a Block Parent. Ben might even get to see a banana slug. I might finally learn to say Tronna and tomaydo and Jell-O and find out if tomato juice really does work on ex-skunkness. I could even get another chance to embarrass Ben with my favourite Buffalo Wing joke. And even if we don't go, we'll always know that we could.

It's sort of OK. And maybe I've missed them all, the people we walked away from so easily. The ones who can find it in their hearts to forgive me for being so irritably superior. Like no-one else ever took a gap year, like we are somehow clever. I love them really. I feel a party coming on.

GLOSSARY

A Transatlantic Lexicon

One of the more unexpected aspects of moving from the UK to Canada was the language barrier. Not mine, everyone else's. We Brits know all about trunks and hoods, candy and cookies etc. from American TV and films. However, according to the kind Canadians who sampled these chapters before publication, there are one or two unfathomable mysteries to unravel. Not only should I should supply a picture of Crystal Tipps, we require a slang glossary. It's mainly for the use of Canadian readers, although Brits may find it mildly entertaining.

A4:   The standard metric paper size for letters and business.

Anorak: An unfashionable version of parka much favoured by train-spotters.

The Archers: The UK's longest running radio soap. It began shortly after World War Two and is still going strong. Its fans are deemed a little odd. You can hear it over the internet now at www.bbc.co.uk/radio4/archers try it, it's fab.

The Beano:	A UK children's comic, much enjoyed by small boys.
Ben Nevis Race:	Ben Nevis is the UK's highest mountain. Every September a bunch of stalwart hill runners race up it and down again. It takes the leaders about an hour and a half.
Blagging:	Stealing, scrounging, smooth talking your way into something you don't deserve.
Blubbing:	Crying.
Bod:	Short for body, just a general reference to a person.
Boffins:	Terribly clever scientificy chaps.
Boot sale:	Garage sale. Not everyone has a garage so loads of you get together to sell thing out of your car boot. (Boot: Trunk.)
British Rail:	Changes of season stop the UK rail network on a regular basis. According to British Rail the weather is generally to blame. Leaves on the line, the wrong sort of rain and the wrong sort of snow all viciously conspire to cause mayhem every year.
Caff:	The cockney pronunciation for café, used to denote a bit of a downmarket version.
Cathedral cities:	In the UK a town can only be a city if it has a cathedral, otherwise it takes an act of parliament to break the rules.

Chemist: A pharmacy or drugstore and the pharmacist who works therein.

Collywobbles: As it sounds really, feeling a bit queasy and wobbly.

Crystal Tipps: Here she is. With her dog Alistair she graced UK children's TV in the 70s:

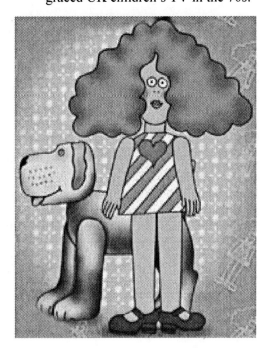

CV: Resume, it's short for Curriculum Vitae which is Latin for 'course of life'. There now, you were expecting a light-hearted read and we're studying Latin. Cripes! (Cripes!: sort of gosh! Or Blimey! Or Holy Hannah Banana! Which doesn't work in an English accent.)

Dobbing:	Well according to my dictionary, this one's Australian …to tell tales or inform on.
Dual carriageway:	Any road where the lanes are divided down the middle by a central reservation. (Central reservation: median.)
Fortnight:	Two weeks. Fourteen nights… geddit?
Garden:	Back (or front) yard, the place you put plants is your flowerbed.
Gobsmacked:	Sort of flabbergasted.
Gormless:	A bit dim.
Guy Fawkes:	The UK sets off its fireworks on November the fifth to commemorate the discovery of loads of gunpowder under the House of Commons, along with Guy Fawkes and his plans to do away with the government of the day. Honestly!
Have I Got News for You:	A popular satirical TV quiz show.
Heath Robinson:	A British cartoonist who drew fantastical gadgets for accomplishing the simplest of tasks. He is now an adjective.
Hinge and Bracket:	A British comedy double-act.
Jobsworth:	The sort of person who wears a uniform in order to be as unhelpful as possible. Whatever is required, it is 'more 'n my job's worth' to oblige.
Juggernaut:	A huge lorry. (Lorry: A truck.)
Jumpers:	Sweaters, not some sort of overall.

Knickers:	Panties, nothing at all to do with odd knee-length trousers. (Trousers: Pants.)
Marigolds:	The brand name for household rubber gloves, like calling bleach Javex (that one had me puzzled for weeks).
Mind The Gap:	Synonymous with the London Underground. There used to just be signs but nowadays there are recorded messages too. They remind you to Mind The Gap whenever you step off a train. Toronto's signs are a lot more helpful than London's though, they show a little person falling between the train and the platform. Londoners have to be careful entirely without the aid of a diagram. Maybe this is why the message has changed in recent years to 'Mind the Gap between the Train and the Platform'. I prefer the pictorial version.
Naff:	A bit inferior really.
Nappy:	Diaper.
NHS:	National Health Service. We love it because it's free and moan about it because it's under funded.
NSPCC:	National Society for the Prevention of Cruelty to Children.
Off Licence:	Or 'offy', the place you buy alcohol to take home. Years ago, before every supermarket and corner shop sold booze, some pubs had a little shop attached that was licensed to sell sealed bottles for off-site consumption.

Pavement:	Now let's get this clear once and for all. The pavement is the bit you walk on. Cars drive on the tarmac and sidewalks happen in movies.
Quid:	Slang for a pound. Think 'buck'.
Rounders:	A children's playground game, a bit like baseball without armour.
Skiving:	Slyly avoiding as much work as possible.
Sleeping policeman:	Speed bump.
Spiv:	The flashy, overdressed guy who can always get stuff on the black market for you.
Takes the Biscuit:	Tops everything else. A biscuit (biccie) is a cookie, not a scone.
Test Match:	Cricket. International Test Matches last 4-5 days and are a great way to while away a long weekend doing nothing.
Tuck box:	A boarding school ritual, this is where you hide your sweets and chocs.
Vest:	An undershirt, the sleeveless thing that goes on top is a waistcoat.
Wheeze:	A really great idea.
Wombles:	Another 1970s children's TV series, the Wombles all had names picked from a world atlas i.e. Great Uncle Bulgaria, Orinoco and of course, Tobermory.

About the Author

Carolyn has been a psychologist, a paramedic, a proofreader and several other things, not all of them beginning with P. She began writing the day she decided to try and see the world...doing both just to find out if she could. Parts of this book appear in the Rough Guides' third *Women Travel* anthology, an event which quite turned her head.

Born and bred in London, England, Carolyn and her son now live permanently back in Kitchener, Ontario. They run a B&B there which they share with sundry pets and call heaven. Carolyn is currently working on the tale of how that came about, which is at least as odd as this story of her first love affair with Canada.

Printed in the United States
42971LVS00001B/111